Nursing in General Practice

Nursing in General Practice

A foundation text

Edited by

Sarah Luft and *Milly Smith*

Senior Lecturers in Health Studies
School of Health Sciences
University of Wolverhampton, UK

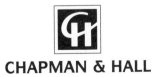

CHAPMAN & HALL

London · Glasgow · Weinheim · New York · Tokyo · Melbourne · Madras

Published by Chapman & Hall, 2–6 Boundary Row, London SE1 8HN

Chapman & Hall, 2–6 Boundary Row, London SE1 8HN, UK

Blackie Academic & Professional, Wester Cleddens Road, Bishopbriggs, Glasgow G64 2NZ, UK

Chapman & Hall GmbH, Pappelallee 3, 69469 Weinheim, Germany

Chapman & Hall Inc., One Penn Plaza, 41st Floor, New York NY 10119, USA

Chapman & Hall Japan, Thomson Publishing Japan, Hirakawacho Nemoto Building, 6F, 1-7-11 Hirakawa-cho, Chiyoda-ku, Tokyo 102, Japan

Chapman & Hall Australia, Thomas Nelson Australia, 102 Dodds Street, South Melbourne, Victoria 3205, Australia

Chapman & Hall India, R. Seshadri, 32 Second Main Road, CIT East, Madras 600 035, India

Distributed in the USA and Canada by Singular Publishing Group Inc., 4284 41st Street, San Diego, California 92105

First edition 1994

© 1994 Chapman & Hall

Typeset in 10/12pt Palatino by Mews Photosetting, Beckenham, Kent
Printed in Great Britain by Page Bros, Norwich.

ISBN 0 412 49840 5   1 56593 187 4 (USA)

A catalogue record for this book is available from the British Library

Library of Congress Catalog Card Number 93-74435

∞ Printed on permanent acid-free text paper, manufactured in accordance with ANSI/NISO Z39.48–1992 and ANSI/NISO Z39.48–1984 (Permanence of Paper).

Contents

Contributors

Alison Allcock RGN, FPCert, ATCDip, Diploma in Office Administration, Practice Nurse/Practice Manager, South London.

Ann Hoskins MB, BCH, BAO, MCommH, MFPHM, Public Health Physician, Liverpool Health Authority.

Sarah Luft BSc(Hons), RGN, NDN, Senior Lecturer in Health Sciences, University of Wolverhampton.

Jacqueline Mansfield RGN, QN, DNT, MA, BA, DipN(Lond), Senior Lecturer in Health Studies, Nottingham Trent University.

David Seedhouse BSc(Hons), PhD, Senior Lecturer in Medical Ethics, University of Auckland, New Zealand.

Milly Smith MSc, RGN, QN, Senior Lecturer in Health Sciences, University of Wolverhampton.

Kevin Snee MBChB, MRCGP, MSc, MFPHM, Public Health Physician, Sefton Health Authority.

Colin Stevenson MA, BM, BCh, MRCGP, MFPHM, Consultant in Public Health Medicine, West Midlands Regional Health Authority.

Monica Tettersell BSc(Hons), PGCE, RGN, RSCN, HVDip, DPSN, Nurse Advisor, Birmingham Family Health Service.

Preface

This book will support the developments in general practice by introducing subjects that influence health care. Although the term **practice nurse** is used throughout the text, **community health care nurse** could equally apply as the editors recognize that much of the material covered is valuable to any nurse who works in the discipline of community health.

Health itself is multifaceted and the contents of this book have been carefully chosen to serve as an introduction to areas of health care that are likely to be new to the majority of readers. The chapters therefore can be viewed as a comprehensive text but each is sufficiently detailed to accommodate a specific framework for its subject area that should provide the basis for competent working knowledge. Hopefully readers will feel inspired to build on the work in these chapters and there is a wealth of specialized and detailed knowledge available in the colleges of higher education, nursing, medical and public libraries that provides material for further reading.

It is not the intention of this book to cover the role and function of nurses working in general practice or discuss clinical aspects of care. These issues are well covered in other texts and it is not possible or necessarily desirable to cover everything in one book.

About this book

CHAPTER 1 HOW SOCIAL POLICY INFLUENCES HEALTH

The major spur for the developments in practice nursing
may have appeared to come from growth within the practice,
but the changes in general practice were first instigated
by policy initiatives from central government. The end of
the 1980s and beginning of the 1990s saw a spate of major
health and social services initiatives that were introduced
through government dicta. Eventually the outcome of each
policy influences the level of patient/client care and this is
where practice nursing also feels the impact. Practice nurses
need to be aware of health policy issues as they influence the
ways in which general practice services respond to the provision of health care.

This chapter presents information on government health
strategies and policies that influence community care. It is
deliberately critical: issues are presented in their official context
and are analysed for the hidden agenda, the intention being
to sharpen awareness between the stated ideal and the reality
of the policy implementation.

CHAPTER 2 LIFESTYLE INFLUENCES ON CLIENT HEALTH

Health is a relative term which very much depends on each
individual's perceptions and these perceptions are coloured
by many influences, some of which are directly associated with
the society in which we live. This chapter explores some of
the aspects of society that either advantage or disadvantage
the individual. The purpose of this exploration is to create

an awareness among practice nurses of the power that is wielded by influences over which the individual has very little control. Sometimes health professionals can be more effective in their work with a wider understanding of the facts that confuse and compound health issues.

CHAPTER 3 MANAGING HEALTH CARE IN GENERAL PRACTICE

The policy initiatives that enhance the role of practice nurses are also the ones that increase demands on expertise. Though this book does not deal with clinical issues it does consider aspects of managing care. Efficient organization is paramount where work is complex and demands are high and a sound understanding of management principles contributes to the smooth running of the system. Acquisition of basic management skills can not only be time and energy saving but can facilitate happy working relationships. Management skills tend to be undervalued as nurses often fail to appreciate just how much they are used in a routine day. Principles of management are found in all aspects of nursing care.

To be effective in a demanding role it is helpful to have an appreciation of basic management techniques. These are not only the skills of organization that ensure the smooth running of the nursing workload. They are also issues associated with providing a quality service, with keeping staff motivated and progressive. The skills associated with teamwork and leadership are areas of rapid growth but for most people they need to be acquired and do not occur naturally. The issues that are drawn upon in this chapter will help the practice nurse to integrate the new and challenging aspects of the role.

CHAPTERS 4 AND 5 EPIDEMIOLOGY

The state of health and ill health in populations is constantly changing. Health professionals must be able to respond to that change and strive to provide appropriate services. The practice nurse as a part of the general practice team has an important role to play in this area and must be able to acquire the necessary skills that facilitate the collection of this epidemiological information.

For many nurses the concept of epidemiology can be a difficult one to grasp but the subject area is very relevant for all nurses who work in the community. The editors have therefore decided that two chapters should be devoted to this subject in order to allow for the introduction and consolidation of new knowledge.

Chapter 4 clearly outlines the content covered and is particularly valuable in that it allows the reader to determine the different aspects that are contained within the discipline of epidemiology. The reader may then choose to concentrate on one or more of these areas initially and build up the total picture over a period of time. This chapter provides a source of reference, enabling the reader to easily find and reread specific topics as and when they are required.

Acquiring knowledge of the practice population demonstrates the value of an understanding of epidemiology for community health care nurses and **Chapter 5** builds on the basic understanding of epidemiology in that some of the pertinent information is reinforced by further analysis and application.

CHAPTER 6 NEEDS AND THE TRULY REFLECTIVE NURSE

This provocative chapter is written by a philosopher who sets out to challenge the readers to examine their understanding of need. Many nurses have not had the opportunity to study philosophy or to consider how philosophical thinking can relate to health. The philosophy of health is now becoming a part of many nurse education programmes and this chapter introduces the reader to a perspective on health which hitherto may not have been addressed. The concept of need is high on various agendas today and Dr Seedhouse offers the opportunity to explore the ways in which a practice nurse may view this concept. The nature of the subject demands that the reader thinks about the ideas and propositions; this can be done through self-reflection but the subject area acts as a basis for continuing debate and therefore is good to share with others.

CHAPTER 7 THE DYNAMICS OF PRACTICE NURSING

This chapter assesses the current state of nursing knowledge. It helps nurses to gain a deeper understanding of their art, which in turn helps them to shape the future of nursing. The chapter concentrates on practice nursing and analyses the position of the nurse within the general practice team. The practice nurse is encouraged to develop a concept of the role and to utilize the ideas generated in order to take a holistic approach to practice nursing and influence the changes and developments that are occurring.

CHAPTER 8 PRACTICE NURSING: PROFESSION OR OCCUPATION?

To make a real contribution to the work of the practice and realize the potential of nursing within general practice, there is a need for the nurse to understand nursing. It is sometimes difficult to consider the contribution that nursing makes because it can be wrapped up in the whole parcel of health care. Nurses and nursing do have something unique to offer within health care but identifying this uniqueness first demands that the nurse explores the identity of nursing. Understanding the position of nursing today and its evolution, particularly in relation to medicine, is helpful to working in a multidisciplinary team. Until nurses truly establish their own identity within the practice team they will continue to be misused and underused. Full contributions from nurses often come about when the nurses take a positive approach and offer ideas and suggestions.

Examination of the concept of the professional nurse is a useful way of determining what nursing is and what it ought to be. The history of nursing has left it with many legacies that remain influential to this day. It has influenced the development of nursing and accounts for the position that nursing holds in relation to other health professions. To appreciate the

most effective ways to take nursing forward, it is necessary
to know what stage of professionalization has been reached
and which factors have been influential in shaping the road
that nursing has taken.

The Editors hope that this text will be a valuable resource for
nurses working within general practice and that it will help
to promote awareness of some of the wider issues that
influence health in society today.

How social policy influences health

Jacqueline Mansfield

INTRODUCTION

Everyone in Britain today expects to be healthy. If by some unfortunate chance they become ill or have a disability they expect to have access to free health care. If they find themselves without financial support, perhaps due to unemployment, illness or old age, they expect to get a state pension if they have paid their 'stamp' or social security benefit if they have not.

This chapter will explain how we in Britain have come to hold these expectations by describing the health and welfare policies that have enabled this level of confidence to develop. It will also discuss how these policies are shaped by political ideologies and processes.

The focus of the chapter is health and health policies. Health in this context is defined as the absence of illness or disease and health care as that care that enables an individual to maintain health within this narrow definition; thus the health policies described are those which relate directly to health care delivery.

However, health policy is just one aspect of social policy. The links between ill health and poverty have been identified time and again by historians, policy makers, social science researchers, health care professionals and by the people themselves. Poverty is the underlying cause of much ill health so this chapter will look at state provision (i.e. the provision of social security) for alleviating poverty.

The chapter is divided into three sections. The first section consists of a discussion of the ideological stances of the major political parties which determine policies and the political processes which shape policy decisions. This is followed by a section examining the introduction of the Welfare State in Britain and the development of health and social security provision up to 1979. The final section concentrates on the impact on health and social security provision of the Thatcher governments of 1979 to 1991.

As a starting point a clarification of the meaning of the term 'social policy' could be helpful. According to Hill, social policy usually includes the areas of social security, the personal social services and health (Hill, 1988). Social policy in this context is seen as the policy of welfare. He then adds that those policies that are classed as 'social' are not the only ones that make a contribution to welfare and that public policy should be viewed as a whole with interlocking and interconnecting elements. Even those policies that are classed as 'social' 'should not be interpreted as if they are the only ones that have the welfare of the public in mind' (p. 4).

Hill goes on to discuss the relationship of social and economic policy and the ratio of welfare to other spending as percentages of the gross domestic product (GDP). He emphasizes that expenditure on social policy must compete with other demands on the budget such as spending on defence. It is only a relatively secure nation state such as Britain that can devote a large proportion of its income to welfare policies. A nation at war, whether within or without its own boundaries, may have very different priorities.

Therefore, when discussing social policy it is also important to consider economic policy as there is often no clear distinction between the two. It is frequently impossible to identify what is strictly economic and what is social in terms of public policy. Weale suggests that it is more helpful to approach the study of social policy from this broad perspective.

We should define social policy not in terms of a specific range of policies or institutions, but rather in terms of a specific set of dimensions of individual welfare, to which a varying range of policy instruments and institutions are relevant.

(Weale, 1983; p. 4)

The relevance to practice nurses of social policy probably lies most directly in knowledge of specifics such as welfare benefits and health care delivery in relation to the needs of their clients. However, to make sense of this specific knowledge it is important to understand the wider issues, 'the dimensions of individual welfare', and also how policy is formulated and why some policy decisions are made and not others. An understanding of the political ideologies of the government in power will help here.

In addition, patient/client advocacy is an area of role development for nurses and practice nurses are no exception. A knowledge of political processes and policy formation could be a useful tool in taking forward an issue on behalf of an individual client or group of clients. Also an understanding of social and economic policies and their constraints could enable the development of an argument that has weight and credibility.

THE POLICY PROCESS, DEMOCRACY
AND POLITICAL IDEOLOGIES

Since the middle of the seventeenth century Britain has enjoyed political stability which has allowed the growth of a strong nation state. Following the restoration of the monarchy in 1659, Parliament, the monarchy and the populace have lived more or less in harmony with the sovereign as the nominal head and the Prime Minister as the actual leader of the state. The political culture of Britain is predominantly one of acceptance by the electorate of the active process of regulating and directing society; in other words, the process of government.

This of course is a very broad generalization. There have been instances of rebellion against the government since that time; currently one example can be seen in Ireland where, following the secession of Southern Ireland from British rule, those people of Northern Ireland who are sympathetic to the republican cause have continued to deny the legitimacy of the British state. Britain, in order to maintain government in

Northern Ireland, has had to rely heavily on coercion through a series of rules and punishments. These have been imposed on the population by the government through their agents of control – the police, the armed forces and the judiciary.

The authority of a state is dependent on the amount of legitimacy it is afforded by the people; that is, the extent to which the people accept the right of the state to govern. In societies where the degree of legitimacy is small the political system is very unstable, revolutions and coups are common and social policy is almost non-existent. Order is maintained through coercion and fear of punishment but an ethos of lawlessness is evident. Many countries of the developing world suffer from this syndrome, as do some of those of the former Eastern Bloc since the collapse of communism.

However in Britain as a whole in recent years, despite political unrest and civil disobedience in Northern Ireland and

> Despite evidence of growing political volatility, of declining public deference to government, the break with elements of consensus government, the curtailment of trade union rights . . . there has been no real threat of a breakdown of liberal, democratic government and limited interest in major constitutional reforms.
>
> *(Pierson, 1991; p. 161)*

The Prime Minister heads the government which consists of members elected to the House of Commons to represent 'the common people' and the peers of the realm who sit in the House of Lords either as a birth right or as a reward for political service. Power to govern and to create policy rests with the House of Commons, the real power of the House of Lords having been effectively curtailed in 1911.

The British system is one of government by democratic control with suffrage extended to the majority of people over the age of 18 (the exceptions being criminals, the insane and peers of the realm). Weale identifies that

> Democracy allows scope for the free competition of ideas in the solution to collective problems . . . and provides a set of procedures in which there is recognition of the equality of the person.
>
> *(Weale, 1983; p. 179)*

A simplistic view is that Britain is a democracy governed by elected representatives who respond to the wishes of their respective electorates. But this is by no means the whole story. In effect, though Members of Parliament are elected, the electorate is not an homogeneous group so responding to the collective wishes of the electorate is an impossible task.

The number of people who vote for the elected candidate is less than the total number who vote, which in turn is more than likely to be less than the total of people who could vote. Consequently the elected member may be representing only a very small proportion of the electorate.

What happens in fact is that the candidate represents the political party of which he/she is a member and it is for that party or for the policies of that party as identified in its manifesto that the electorate votes. Even so, as those proponents of proportional representation will be aware, the party gaining the most seats in the House of Commons and thus overall government control is not necessarily the party which attracted the most votes.

Given that a representative democracy can never be truly representative the question that must be addressed is why the current electoral system continues to work in Britain.

Perhaps the answer lies partly in the electoral system itself, where each government must seek re-election after five years in office. This means that the politicians must remain in touch with the electorate and policies must be continually modified in order to retain popular support, one feature of democratic politics. However, to be truly democratic the system must also include universal suffrage, state action governed by law not by individuals and must emphasize civil liberties such as freedom of speech, freedom of movement and freedom of worship, all of which are characteristics of the British system of social order.

Democracy is dependent on the state being free to respond not only to the political demands of the electorate as a whole but also to the demands of specific pressure (interest) groups. Interest group activity can supply the state with information between one election and the next which will allow the decision makers opportunity to weigh up the various demands. Thus pressure groups can inform the development of future policy. Democracy is essentially 'pluralist' in character with politicians involved in continuous negotiation and compromise between themselves and a variety of groups representing different elements of society.

The policy making process within democratic pluralism can be seen as a system which depends on inputs, throughputs and outputs. This is described very clearly by Ham (1982) in his analysis of work done by Easton (1953). This analysis considers that inputs consist of demands and supports; demands are made by the electorate, interest groups and other external agencies and supports include the actions of the electorate such as voting, obedience to the law and payment of taxes. Throughput involves decision making and all that that implies, described by Ham as the conversion process. The result of the conversion process is the output – the decisions that are made and the resulting policies. (Outcomes, on the other hand, are the effects of these policies on the electorate.) Feedback is allowed for within this process as outputs are fed back to influence future inputs into the system.

The throughput or conversion process is formalized within Parliament itself using the mechanisms of Green and White Papers for wide consultation with the electorate in general and interest groups in particular and through the agency of various committees such as the select committees which have the power to consult specific interested parties and make recommendations to the government.

Royal Commissions may be set up to enquire into and report on a specific area. These reports tend to be known by the surname of the chairperson; the Briggs Report (or more correctly, the Report of the Committee on Nursing 1972) was chaired by Lord Briggs and is one example which is of particular relevance to nursing.

However, in recent years Royal Commissions have been abandoned in favour of government initiated reviews and enquiries, again of specific areas. These are carried out by small teams of people appointed by the government with a remit to report within a given time, often six months, as opposed to Royal Commissions which were well known for the thoroughness of their reviews but also for the large numbers of people involved and the length of time between receiving the commission and the government receiving the report.

What must also be remembered when analysing the policy making process is that power is shared between ministers and civil servants with continuity being provided by the latter. This is perhaps one of the stabilizing features of the British parliamentary system and the one which enables the process of government to proceed smoothly despite changes within the government and changes of government following general elections. It also begs the question – where does the ultimate power lie?

The policy making process is standard to all British governments whatever their political persuasion but the policies produced will be influenced by the ideology of the party in power. For example, all political parties in Britain subscribe to the principle of a welfare state but the degree of commitment to state welfare differs as the policies of each party show.

As a very broad generalization (and descriptions of political parties must be broad to allow for the many variations of ideology within the spectrum of political views), the ideology of the Conservative Party is based on liberalism which believes in the right of the individual to feedom of choice. Each person is seen as a rational being capable of making rational decisions who is responsible for his/her own actions. The role of the state is passive, limited and neutral – a minimal framework only. Welfare provision is at a basic minimum in order to allow the individual freedom to choose alternatives to state welfare for himself and his dependants.

Within the ideology of liberalism two distinct strands can be identified – the liberal collectivists and the anticollectivists or New Right. The two strands represent moderate and extreme views of liberalism respectively.

Typical policy preferences of liberal collectivists include those which emphasize the value of individual initiative and freedom for private enterprise with little state intervention except in the area of maintaining law and order, which is seen as high priority. Originally liberalism stressed freedom of the individual as the ultimate goal but by the mid 1900s the emphasis, particularly in economic policy, changed 'to be associated with a readiness to rely primarily on the state rather than on private voluntary arrangements to achieve objectives as desirable. The catchwords became welfare and equality rather than freedom'

(Potter, 1982). It was this change of emphasis that allowed for compromise and consensus between the main political parties over the post-Second World War policies and legislation that introduced the Welfare State.

The ideology of the New Right (sometimes called anti-collectivism) is a regeneration of the original free market philosophy postulated by Adam Smith in his book *The Wealth of Nations* written in 1776. It extends the idea of freedom of the individual to freedom of the market and emphasizes the value to the economy of market forces and competition. The state plays little or no part in regulating the economy; this is the function of the market with its laws of supply and demand.

Followers of this ideology are opposed to the Welfare State on the grounds that it aims for equality of outcome and redistribution of wealth. These are seen to be harmful to the growth of productivity and efficiency and therefore impediments to market processes. The concept of equality is an anathema to some anticollectivists but they accept that there may be a need for minimal state provision of welfare in exceptional circumstances.

Otherwise the state is seen to have little part to play in the provision of welfare, especially in giving economic support. Exponents of the New Right, including Thatcher, believe that the state should return the responsibility for self-care to the individual and that includes the responsibility for making financial provision to meet the common hazards of life such as sickness, unemployment and old age.

The second very broad political ideology present in British politics today is that of the branch of socialism pursued by the British Labour Party and to some extent the Social Democratic Party and which is an almost direct antithesis to the ideology of the New Right.

Within this philosophy the state is seen as having a very positive and supportive role, especially to those in need. At the same time it is expansionist in that, in order to deal with the complex problems of society, a large number of state controlled organizations need to be set up to monitor the welfare of the people. The term 'Nanny State' has been coined to describe the policies enacted within this framework, particularly in relation to the setting up of the Welfare State.

However, despite differing political ideologies, for much of the lifetime of the Welfare State British politics have kept firmly to the middle ground. The Welfare State was founded on the consensus view of all political parties that what was required in postwar Britain was a system of state welfare provision. This consensus remained as the underlying philosophy until 1979, albeit with increasing dissension. It was only with the Thatcher government of 1979 that consensus finally crumbled to allow real party political differences to surface.

THE DEVELOPMENT OF THE WELFARE STATE

This section is written on the premise that it is only by understanding the history of the Welfare State that the true relevance of its subsequent development becomes apparent.

The two aspects of the Welfare State that will be examined here are health care provision and social security but the reader should bear in mind that other aspects, namely education, housing and employment, also need to be taken into account when analysing the totality of state welfare provision.

In looking at the development of the Welfare State the interdependence of health care and financial provision becomes apparent in that health care delivery has always been dependent on the ability to pay – either by the individual or by the state.

Prior to the NHS Act the burden of payment rested on the individual with some state aid. Following the implementation of the Act the balance shifted; payment for health care became the responsibility of the state but based on the system of insurance contributions made by those in employment. If individuals preferred to pay privately for their health care this was also acceptable though they were still liable for their National Insurance contribution.

Though 1946 is often quoted as the year of the birth of the Welfare State, state involvement in the welfare of the poor can be traced back to the Elizabethan Poor Law Reform Act of 1601 and the subsequent New Poor Law Act of 1834 which are the antecedents of the current social security system. The Elizabethan Poor Law Act, in placing the responsibility for the poor upon each parish, imposed a centrally determined framework on a system of relief which previously had been ad hoc and locally determined. A system of 'out relief', that is the distribution of assistance, cash or kind, to the poor of the parish to enable them to maintain a minimum standard of living, was established. This enabled the poor and destitute to survive but at starvation level. Medical and nursing care, such as it was, was also provided and paid for by the parish at a minimum level.

The system of out relief was tightened up by the New Poor Law Act of 1834 which formed parishes into groups – Poor Law unions – and brought in measures to curb indiscriminate granting of out relief. This Act is notorious for the introduction of the 'workhouse test' and the doctrine of 'less eligibility' where the conditions in workhouses (local authority administered institutions for the destitute) were designed to be such that only the desperate would seek to enter. The system of 'less eligibility' was based on means testing to ensure that those getting state relief were worse off than the poorest worker. (*Oliver Twist* by Charles Dickens gives a contemporary commentary on conditions in the workhouse following the 1834 Act, albeit with a degree of poetic licence.)

In Victorian England, being poor was seen to be the fault of the individual, especially if poverty was caused by unemployment (idleness). This group of people were termed the undeserving (i.e. undeserving of charity) poor. The deserving poor, on the other hand, were those people made poor through no fault of their own – perhaps deserted wives would fall into this category. It might be worth considering whether the notion of deserving and undeserving poor still persists, especially in relation to state social security provision.

War often acts as a stimulus for policy reform, especially social policy, as is clearly demonstrated by public and state response to the Boer War when it was discovered that a large proportion of potential recruits had to be turned down because they were physically unfit. Britain did not perform at all well in this war much to the surprise of the populace and more particularly to the surprise of the politicians. The ultimate result of this poor performance was an examination and subsequent reform of social policy, including the setting up of the school medical and school meals services in 1904. Hill (1988) quotes Fraser in stating

> In that bizarre way which again and again seemed to link imperialism with social reform (sometimes as allies, sometimes as competitors) it seemed to some that Britain would only be able to sustain its Empire if she ensured that the new generation of children, tomorrow's Imperial Army, was properly nourished.
>
> *(Fraser, 1973)*

Poverty was seen as the precursor of much ill health and so an indepth survey of the extant social security mechanisms was undertaken. This eventually led to the enactment by Lloyd George's Liberal Government of the Old Age Pension Act 1908 which gave a means tested, non-contributory benefit and the National Insurance Act 1911 which introduced the insurance principle into British social security legislation for the first time and gave rise to the system of contributory benefits.

Events overtook the social policy reforms of Lloyd George's Liberal Government; the advent of the First World War in 1914 followed by the economic recession of the 1920s and slump of the early 1930s meant that the pace of policy reform slowed. However, there was a growing awareness of social problems, including those of poverty brought about by unemployment and ill health brought about in part by poor housing conditions, also often linked to poverty.

The dominant ideology of the major political parties in the latter part of this period (that is, the 1930s and 1940s) and extending into the postwar years was liberal collectivism and with it a commitment to a system of state provision for welfare. As a measure of this a committee was set up in 1941 under the chairmanship of Sir William Beveridge to enquire into social insurance schemes. The resulting report, Social Insurance and Allied Services 1942 (better known as the Beveridge Report), laid the foundation for the modern welfare state.

In his report Beveridge made a wide-ranging analysis of the social ills of Britain which he described as the five giants of want, indolence, ignorance, squalor and disease. However, he focused his report on the diagnosis of want (poverty) and the impact of this on the lives of the population. He postulated that a substantial proportion of those in poverty were poor because of interruption to or loss of earning power so the main thrust of the report consists of proposals for income maintenance. As a corollary to this he recommended the development of a national health service so that treatment could be offered to minimize interruption in earning power.

As a liberal collectivist Beveridge believed that poverty and insecurity are disfunctional and threatening to capitalist order. Consequently state intervention is necessary in a liberal market economy but at a minimal level (Cutler *et al.*, 1986).

Amongst the Beveridge proposals that were accepted and implemented was one for setting up a system of social security, dominated by compulsory social insurance, the aim of which was to abolish poverty by redistributing income within the wage earning class.

As a consequence the postwar social security system was a universal system of national insurance and was based on contributions made by the worker, his employer and the state. A sufficient level of contribution ensured benefits for sickness, unemployment and old age.

To act as a safety net for those whose contributions were insufficient to enable them to receive benefit a system of non-contributory means tested benefits was introduced, known initially as National Assistance, later as Social Security and currently as Income Support.

Beveridge's proposals and subsequent legislation were based on several assumptions about life in postwar Britain. Firstly there was the assumption of full employment which would ensure that the fiscal gap (the gap between income received by the government through taxes and income expended by the government on benefits) remained small or non-existent. Secondly it was assumed that women would return to caring for children after the war, thus leaving their husbands to earn the family income. A husband and wife were treated as a single unit under Beveridge and it was the husband's income that was crucial, not his wife's. Hence allowances for child support, whilst available to all fathers (not mothers), were minimal in relation to the cost of child care and applied only to the second child and subsequent children. The purpose of family allowance was not to replace the wife's income as she would not be working anyway, but to help with the cost of additional children. It was felt that the father's income was sufficient to cover the cost of the first child.

It is perhaps worth noting that Beveridge's assumptions about family income, though now wildly anachronistic, dominated social security policy up until 1990 when separate taxation for husbands and wives was introduced.

On hindsight and with the benefit of knowledge it is easy to be scathing about the recommendations of the Beveridge Report in relation to social security and to criticize his assumptions about the family but few reports have had as far reaching consequences as this one.

Beveridge based his reforms on an economy where full employment was the expectation. It was impossible for him to foresee the events that were to overtake the economic systems of the world, such as the oil crisis of 1973, the technological revolution which has resulted in increasing unemployment as industry becomes less labour intensive and galloping inflation, again leading to more and more job losses as firms close down; in fact, all the problems that beset Britain's economy today.

Social mores have also changed over time. Today more marriages are ending in divorce, leaving many single parents with state support as their only means of income. Alternatively marriage is not always seen as the essential basis for a relationship into which children are born. The resulting informal liaison can lead to instability of family life, possibly again with an increase in the number of single parents needing state support.

Demographic changes have led to a huge increase in the numbers of people of retirement age who are entitled to state benefit which again could not have been foreseen by Beveridge. However, all these and other changes have led successive governments to assess and reassess the social security system which in turn has led to constant tinkering with benefit and contribution levels in an attempt to meet needs and balance the books. A major reform of the social security system did take place in 1986 to 'tidy it up' but even Thatcher's best efforts were not able to override Beveridge's original concept of a system of national insurance leading to universal benefits and supplemented by a top-up system of means tested benefits. To date state involvement in welfare still predominates even in a free market economy.

The system of state provision of health care, the National Health Service, also owes its rationalization and development, but not its origins, to Beveridge. The early origins of health care provision rest with religious orders and charities. Certainly by the mid to late nineteenth century, the time of massive industrial expansion and a commensurate increase in ill health, health care for the sick poor tended to fall to the remit of the charitable organizations rather than the state. Those who could afford a small weekly financial outlay paid into friendly societies to insure against sickness and meet the cost of health care.

Institutional care pre-NHS was divided between the voluntary hospitals (so called because they existed as a result of voluntary support) and the municipal Poor Law infirmaries, which had developed from the workhouse system as institutions to care for the chronic sick and elderly infirm.

As an alternative to institutional care, and especially to meet the needs of those who could not afford to pay, many of the large voluntary hospitals operated dispensaries, the equivalent of outpatient departments today, where the poor could seek advice, medication and often food and clothing in an emergency.

General practitioners tended to work from singlehanded practices and because GPs relied on private patients to make up their income (capitation fees paid from National Health Insurance were very low) they were concentrated in middle class urban communities. To enter general practice the newcomer had to purchase the 'good will' of the retiring doctor, which frequently included his house as well as his surgery. The price of the practice often depended on the number of private patients – the more that were 'on the books', the higher the price – so many young doctors began their careers in general practice heavily in debt.

For the patient the problem of paying for health care was very real. Anecdotal evidence suggests that the doctor was not always called when necessary because the patient could not afford to pay. On the other hand many GPs waived their fees if they were aware of extreme hardship.

By 1948 a variety of systems were in place to help with payment for treatment, for example National Health Insurance which was introduced in 1911. The Act required each worker to pay a weekly contribution out of his wage towards the cost of sickness benefit. This contribution would be matched by equal contributions from the employer and the state for the purpose of paying for treatment by general practitioners. (Hospital care was outside the scheme and was provided either by the voluntary hospitals, still dependent on private funding, or local authority municipal infirmaries, as the old Poor Law hospitals had become.)

General practitioners were very resistant to the National Insurance scheme, initially fearing state control and thus loss of freedom and, with state paid salaries, loss of income. They capitulated eventually when the government agreed that payment would be based on a capitation system rather than a salary. Also the scheme would be administered by independent insurance committees or 'panels', not by local authorities (Ham, 1982). Nevertheless capitation fees were relatively low.

Prior to the NHS Act some preventative services were available, provided by the local authority, such as the school health service, child health clinics, domiciliary midwifery and health visiting, whereas home nursing services still tended to be run by voluntary organizations.

Health care provision was fragmented, developments had occurred in an ad hoc way with little logic and continuity and state control was patchy and ineffective. However, over the years several reports had been initiated by various governments, each of which recommended in essence the development of systems of state controlled comprehensive hospital and primary health care services. Eventually, when the time was right, the Beveridge Report (1942) proposed the development of a national health service. This proposal was accepted and in 1944 a Green Paper was formulated seeking agreement for the plans from interested parties.

However, just as in 1911 when GPs were resistant to the National Insurance Act, so in 1944 the medical profession as a body expressed extreme disapproval of the report. The BMA acting as a powerful pressure group almost succeeded in killing off the NHS before it had begun. The ensuing fight between the medical profession and the government of the day is now history but the concessions demanded by the doctors and granted by the government before the proposals could be accepted still continue to influence health care delivery. These include independent employment status for doctors, the independent contractor system for GPs, the option of private practice, access to pay beds, etc., all of which are designed to ensure that the medical profession retains control over its income and freedom from central (government) control (Ham, 1982).

What also remains is the struggle for power between the medical profession and the government, as the next section of this chapter will show.

Eventually, despite medical opposition – from hospital consultants, not GPs – the National Health Services Act 1946 was passed and the NHS launched on the 'appointed day' in 1948. Its remit, as stated in the Act, is

> To promote the establishment . . . of a comprehensive health service designed to secure improvement in the physical and mental health of the people of England and Wales, and the prevention, diagnosis and treatment of illness, and for that purpose, to provide or secure the effective provision of services in accordance with the following provision of this Act. The service so provided shall be free of charge, except where any provision of this Act expressly provides for the making and recovery of charges.
>
> *(DHSS, 1946)*

The administrative structure of the NHS was based on the pattern of health care delivery that had been in operation previously though some new bodies were introduced. The resultant (tripartite) structure consisted of three branches – GP services administered by executive councils, community health services administered by local authorities and hospital services administered either by boards of governors or hospital management committees, depending on the type of hospital.

Executive councils

The branch that bore the closest resemblance to what had happened before was that which contained the general practitioner services. These, under the Act, were joined with the dentists, the opticians and the pharmacists and administered by executive councils which replaced insurance committees.

There was an exhortation in the Act to build health centres but this was not heeded at that time. However, by the mid 1960s a shift had occurred in the thinking surrounding the provision of health centres. The government of the day spearheaded the change by introducing the Doctor's Charter in 1966 which made money available to GPs over and above capitation fees, some of which went into the development of health centres and group practices.

This development also led to the development of primary health care teams, with local authority employed community nurses working from health centres 'attached' to GPs rather than covering geographical patches as had been the previous system. Some GPs employed practice nurses to run their treatment rooms. Interest in the development of group practices intensified and by the mid 1970s GPs were beginning to employ practice managers and deputizing services were introduced. The increase in property values also led many GPs to purchase rather than rent their practice premises.

Local authority services

Local authority services included community nurses, i.e. district nurses, health visitors and school nurses, maternity and child welfare clinics, health education, vaccination and immunization, ambulances and a range of environmental and personal social services all under the control of the Medical Officer of Health and totally separate from family health services administered by executive councils.

Hospital services

The third branch, equally separate from the other two, was the hospital sector, further subdivided into teaching hospitals under boards of governors and non-teaching hospitals administered by regional hospital boards and hospital management committees.

From the beginning the NHS had financial difficulties. The optimistic estimates made in 1946 that the need for health care would decline as the nation's health improved were soon seen to be unrealistic and calls for extra resources became commonplace. The tripartite structure of the NHS grew into an administrative nightmare and the lack of communication between the three branches became increasingly difficult, particularly for GPs and their consultant colleagues, leading to a widening of the gap between general practice and hospital specialisms.

Of course this did not happen overnight; in fact it took some 20 years or so for the need for reorganization of the NHS to be appreciated, particularly in relation to the cumbersome tripartite structure. Eventually, following extensive consultation, a new structure was devised and the National Health Services Reorganization Act (DHSS, 1973) came into operation on April 1st 1974).

The aims of this Act were threefold, the first of which was to unify the health services under one authority. This in fact was only partially achieved as general practitioners remained independent contractors but were now contracting through family practitioner committees, as the executive councils had now become.

The second aim was to improve co-ordination between health authorities and local government services. Consequently the new area health authorities introduced by the Act were intended to have similar boundaries to local authorities. (Local authorities were to retain control over the personal social services.)

The third aim was to improve the management structure. Nursing management structures had already been rationalized by the Salmon and Mayston Reports of 1966 and 1968 respectively and the 'cogwheel' reports had led to similar developments for medical staff but the 1974 reorganization of the NHS was intended to build on these developments and to include concepts of multidisciplinary team working and consensus management.

The new NHS structure comprised 15 regional health authorities and 90 area health authorities, most of which were further subdivided into a number of district health authorities. Family practitioner committees were at area level and as a totally new concept, community health councils – 'the patient's watchdogs' – were introduced at district level.

This structure did not remain popular for very long. Criticisms included those relating to the cost of the reorganization, the problems of communication between region, area and district and the delay in taking decisions. Overall there was a feeling of unease at an administrative system which was top heavy with administrators and consisted of too many tiers. The Royal Commission on the NHS (DHSS, 1979), chaired by Lord Merrison, confirmed this unease and recommended, amongst many other things, that one tier of the NHS should be removed, which Thatcher did in the 1982 restructuring of the NHS.

The dominant political theme throughout these years has been continuing commitment to and consensus over the Welfare State. Wicks has described the development of the Welfare State as occurring in three stages: 1942 to 1951 – the years of construction; 1951 to the mid 1960s – the years of development and growth; and mid 1960s to 1979 – the years of anxiety and uncertainty (Wicks, 1987). The fourth stage – 1979 to 1992 – will probably be known in time to come as the years of the internal market, as the next section of this chapter will show.

THE THATCHER YEARS

1979 has been described as a watershed in British politics; the end of consensus and the beginning of very real and obvious differences in the political stances of the major parties, not least over the Welfare State. 1979 saw the election of the Conservative government under Thatcher. One result of this is that every area of social policy now bears the stamp of Thatcherism; no area has remained untouched.

Thatcher and health policy

Three areas of the health policies of the Thatcher government will be examined here: managerial accountability, the NHS and Community Care Act (DHSS, 1990c) and the changing focus of health care delivery from curative to preventative care.

Since the end of World War Two and the introduction of state medicine, there have been many improvements in the health of the nation (albeit with noticeable exceptions – see Townsend and Davidson, 1988). The NHS is an undoubted success but arguably it has also become a victim of its own success, having grown into a monster ever hungry for resources.

From its earliest days the NHS has become more and more expensive as demands for health care have increased. Advances in technology have enabled the development of treatment initiatives that were undreamed of in 1948; for example, organ transplants and open heart surgery are now commonplace. The universal availability of advanced medical knowledge, research and technology and the resultant expertise have made the NHS the envy of the world.

Developing medical knowledge has meant the discovery through sophisticated diagnostic testing of 'new' diseases and the consequent searches for a cure. The development of more sophisticated treatments has meant that many people with chronic illness can be helped to live to a greater age than would have once been thought possible; advances in treatment for children with cystic fibrosis is one success story in this area. Consequently the focus of the NHS has changed from treatment of short term, acute illness to maintenance and control of long term chronic disease. The result of new developments and long term care of chronic disease is an increasing demand for appropriate resources – financial and human.

The effect of demographic change also has implications for health care resources. One example of this is the growing number of old people in the population which has increased steadily over the second half of this century and is likely to continue to do so. Old people, especially those over the age of 75 – the 'old old' – are the greatest users of NHS provision of any population group. Harrison states

> The average *per capita* cost of hospital and community health care for the seventy-five years and over group is almost five times that of the national average (that is for all ages) or nine times that of persons of working age.
> *(Harrison, 1988; p. 82)*

Over the years the cost of the NHS had grown exponentially so that the chances of closing the gap between demands and the resources available to meet demands have become less and less possible. Initiatives by successive governments aimed at reducing the gap have been a feature of health policy for many years, almost from the first day of the NHS Act.

In 1979 Thatcher inherited a legacy of a successful, much valued national health service – a national institution – but one which was becoming an increasing nightmare in terms of its demands. In addition there was no real system of accounting for where and how the resources were deployed. Lack of managerial accountability to central government over the use of resources was a feature of the NHS pre-1979, as was the power of the medical profession to command resources in the name of clinical freedom, thus negating accountability. The role of central government seemed to be to supply finance but not to ask questions as to how the money was spent.

Managerial accountability

Problems in this area arose partly as a result of the 1974 NHS reforms which were based on a system of management by consensus. This resulted in decision making processes which were slow, laborious and costly in time and manpower. Consensus demands many meetings and consultations to ensure that all interested parties agree. Accountability for decisions made rests with committees rather than individuals and there is often little incentive to ensure that decisions are implemented.

In 1983 Thatcher appointed a team of four people headed by Sir Roy Griffiths to undertake a management enquiry into the NHS. The resulting Griffiths Report (DHSS, 1983) identified many concerns about the NHS management system. These have been summarized by Harrison as

Individual management accountability could not be located.

The machinery of implementation was generally weak.

There was a lack of orientation towards performance in the service . . . rarely are precise management objectives set . . . clinical evaluation of particular practices is by no means common and economic evaluation of these practices is extremely rare.

There was a lack of concern with the views of consumers of health services.

(Harrison, 1988; p. 68)

Many of the Griffiths recommendations designed to meet the concerns identified were subsequently implemented. The basis for the Griffiths reforms was the replacement of management by consensus with a system of general management, a concept 'borrowed' from the business world. This system vests the ultimate power of decision making and implementation with one individual – the general manager. In the NHS, as general management replaced management by consensus, large, cumbersome management teams were replaced by smaller, 'leaner' management boards which had the remit to get things done and, most importantly, carried accountability for their actions.

Another part of the Griffiths initiative was the introduction of performance related pay and fixed term contracts for senior managers as additional incentive to meet the performance related personal and organizational objectives that they were required to set.

Pre-Griffiths, the Thatcher government had stated that it expected that 'efficiency savings' would be made in the NHS and had developed a system of review and the use of performance indicators to facilitate this. Formal review processes were carried out at regional, district and unit levels using performance indicators to measure local outputs of NHS care delivery and also to compare differences between districts.

Following the Griffiths reforms this system was extended to include clinicians in the form of resource management initiatives which were designed to measure not only outputs but also outcomes of health care delivery.

Harrison (1988) sees that the Griffiths and other government reforms challenged the domination of the medical profession within the NHS in two ways. Firstly aspects of clinical freedom and medical authority were challenged by the appointment of general managers who can veto the traditional power of clinicians on management teams. Secondly the review process had the potential to shift priorities away from prestigious areas such as pioneering surgery towards less prestigious ones such as care of older people, the mentally ill and those with learning difficulties. This threatens the power of consultants to command resources for their acute specialisms. However Harrison concludes that there is little evidence as yet (1988) that the challenge has been successful.

The success of Thatcher's NHS policies for managers in relation to financial accountability and cost containment can be seen. A new 'tougher' breed of manager is now in post, management style is more aggressive and decisions are made on the basis of objectives and implemented with speed. Managers are much more cost conscious and accountable for their actions. Cost cutting exercises are no longer a novelty.

On the other hand many would argue that cost cutting can go too far – pruning a tree of dead wood is healthy but too much pruning can kill it.

NHS and Community Care Act 1990

With this Act a concept new to Britain, that of the internal market, has been introduced into state delivery of health care.

Thatcher, true to her free market, anti-collectivist ideology, introduced this system into the NHS as a means of reducing the costs of health care. She believed that the mechanisms of market forces (economic regulation through competition, supply and demand) would promote efficiency and economy and ensure that the NHS met the needs of the consumer.

In order to achieve this a system of separating out the functions of purchasing and providing care has been introduced (historically all sectors of the NHS have carried out both functions). The purchasers of health care are district health authorities on behalf of their resident populations and family health services authorities and general practitioners on behalf of their practice populations. District health authorities are purchasing a range of services including preventative care based on a health needs assessment, whereas GPs are purchasing episodes of treatment. The providers of health care are the directly managed units, NHS trusts and the private sector.

Under this system purchasing and providing health care is carried out as a contract based business transaction as follows. The purchaser outlines what he wants to buy and the provider furnishes the purchaser with a detailed specification of what he can offer; this will include costs of treatment, staffing costs, etc., quality assurance measures and measures to ensure consumer satisfaction. The specification will also include a mission statement identifying the aims of the provider unit. The purchaser has the power to compare specifications from as many providers as he wishes before deciding on the most appropriate. Thus it is sensible for the provider to ensure that his specification is competitive and attractive to the purchaser. Competition in a market economy ensures that prices are kept down but quality is maintained.

When the purchaser has decided to buy, a contract is drawn up between the two parties. Types of contract include:

- Block contracts when the purchaser agrees to buy a 'block' of care for an identified price; for example, all the hospital care needed by the patients of one GP practice for one year.
- A cost and volume contract, where the purchaser agrees to buy a specified number of episodes of care or procedures at a specified price; for example, 20 hip replacements at £x.
- A cost per case contract issued for an individual case or episode of treatment.

Initially (April 1991) block contracts were the most popular as they are easiest to calculate and administer but as systems have become more sophisticated cost and volume contracts are becoming more popular with providers as they are less risky in economic terms.

Successful contracting depends on many factors including the ability of the provider to set a realistic price and the purchaser to meet the price as promised. When this does not happen bankruptcy can result. So far the government has 'bailed out' units threatened by bankruptcy but whether they are prepared to continue to do this remains to be seen.

Another great change brought about by the NHS and Community Care Act has been the development of NHS trusts. Units within the NHS, on the submission of a satisfactory business plan, have been given government approval to opt out of direct central government control whilst still remaining part of the NHS. It must be stressed here that NHS trusts are still part of the NHS, not privatized businesses. In business terminology a trust is a type of NHS franchise.

Trusts are run as mini businesses, managed by boards of directors headed by a chief executive, within the overall state business of health. As such they have total control over their own resources and power to generate and spend their own income in the best interests of their patients. They also have the power to set terms and conditions of service for all staff. The purpose of this system is to devolve power down to the actual providers of care, thus withdrawing state control (rolling back the frontiers of the state) and introducing competition between units.

In the field of primary health care the principle of trust status is carried out through GP fundholders. GPs, initially with a practice population of 11 000 but now extended to those with a population of 9000, are given the opportunity to opt out from central control to some extent by directly managing a proportion of their budgets (the rest of the budget is controlled by the FHSA). This initiative has led to the development of GP business empires where money gained from income generating activities is ploughed back into the practice to enhance patient services and thus attract more people to register with the GP. GP fundholding practices are run by management teams, a prominent member of which is often the accountant. The advantage of GP fundholding to the practice includes the ability of the GP as a purchaser of care to buy the best service for the practice population which often means the earliest service. The fundholding GP has the power to circumvent waiting lists by buying care from the most appropriate provider and, as a purchaser, to dictate the terms of the contract to some extent.

A fundholding GP from April 1st 1993 can also purchase the services of health authority employed community nurses from the provider unit. Initially the level of service provision must be maintained without virement to the GP budget but eventually any savings made by the GP, perhaps as a result of variations in skill mix, may be used by him/her to purchase additional practice, rather than health authority, staff.

The switch from curative to preventative health care

One feature of the health policies of the Thatcher government has been the shift in focus of health care away from secondary (institutional) and towards primary (community based) health care. This was brought about by many factors, not least perhaps by the growing realization that prevention is cheaper than cure. However, one factor undoubtedly is Britain's membership of the WHO and her consequent commitment to 'health for all by the year 2000'.

In social policy terms this commitment has led to a series of Green and White Papers such as *Promoting Better Health* (DHSS, 1987), *Working for Patients*, (DHSS, 1990a), *The New*

GP Contract (DHSS, 1990b), *The Health of the Nation* (DoH, 1991) and *Health of the Nation: Strategy for Action* (DoH, 1992), all of which carry the government's message in relation to health promotion and prevention of ill health and all of which point up the pivotal role of primary health care in this area.

In these papers the government's strategy for promoting health is spelled out, namely the importance of reducing the high mortality and morbidity from preventable diseases thus 'adding years to life: an increase in life expectancy and reduction in premature death and adding life to years: increasing years lived free from ill health . . .' (DoH, 1992; p. 13). This will be accomplished in many ways, for example by achieving targets for childhood immunization, for cervical cytology, for reduction in incidence of the major causes of mortality. Health education aimed at encouraging life enhancing behaviour and discouraging 'unhealthy' lifestyles is the cornerstone of the strategy.

GPs have the prime role to play in carrying forward the aims of the strategy. The new contract for GPs, which became effective on 1st April 1990, concentrated on health promotion and disease prevention as a formal element of general practice – an explicit rather than an implicit role for GPs. One of the results of this has been a huge increase in the numbers of practice nurses employed (a 60% increase in 1990 alone) to assist GPs in this area. However, a perhaps unexpected consequence of the enthusiasm with which GPs have tackled their health promotion role has been the proliferation in health promotion clinics to the extent that the government has now produced further guidlines relating to the types of clinics that are appropriate and so attract funding and those which are not.

Other conditions of the contract that must be met include an annual health surveillance for those practice patients over the age of 75 who wish for one and a health assessment of all new patients to the practice, again roles usually allotted to the practice nurse.

In addition there has been a rapid increase in computerization in general practice, assisted by an additional government allocation of £24 million in 1990 to allow payments to be made to GPs to buy systems. The use of computers aids in call and recall programmes for immunizations and cervical cytology, for example, but computers in general practice have many other uses (DoH, 1991).

The introduction of the new GP contract was facilitated by the extended powers granted to family health services authorities (FHSAs), as family practitioner services (FPCs) became in 1990. This move was part of the government strategy for improving primary health care as identified in the White Paper *Promoting Better Health* (DHSS, 1987). The extended and strengthened role for FHSAs was implemented in order to enable clearer priorities to be set for the family health services in relation to the rest of the NHS.

In line with the general management principle the cumbersome FPCs with some 30 members were reconstituted to become FHSAs with 11, including appointments from industry and commerce. The administrative framework has been tightened and quality and value for money have become the principal foci for action. Managerial accountability has moved away from central government towards regional health authorities, thus facilitating opportunities for partnership between health authorities and FHSAs, for example in assessing the health needs of the population. In some instances the potential partnerships have become actual.

Currently FHSAs are charged with the responsibility for

... assessing local population needs for family health services, planning services to meet those needs, and managing the contracts of family practitioners, including the targeting of cash-limited funds for general medical practitioners' ancillary staff and premises to areas of greatest need.
(DHSS, 1990b)

In addition the FHSAs are responsible for setting the limit for the allocation of funding for prescriptions to each practice under the indicative prescribing scheme and for monitoring GP fundholding practices.

The role of the FHSA has become one of managing the delivery of family health services whereas previously the focus was very much that of administering contracts. The increasing importance afforded to the FHSA and the introduction of the new GP contract are indications of the importance attached by the government to primary health care but also of their determination to control GPs.

Thatcher has been the first Prime Minister to tackle the doctors and come anywhere near winning. Her victories, though small, have been significant. The concept of clinical freedom has been challenged and doctors are now accountable for the outcomes as well as the outputs of the care they give. GPs have accepted the new contract despite initial threats to resign en masse and are very committed to health promotion to the extent that immunization targets which were once thought to be unrealistic are now being reached or even exceeded. Health education is a significant feature of the service offered by GP practices and most practice premises are now 'user friendly' (the exceptions being some of the London practices where conditions for patients and GPs are amongst the worst in the country). Audit systems are in place together with other quality assurance measures so accountability is easily traced.

However, though the avowed intent of the government is to improve the health of the nation there has been little acknowledgement that an underlying cause of ill health is poverty. Instead the emphasis is on self-help and on improving health by altering behaviour and lifestyle. While these aspects are important there has also to be a recognition that without an infrastructure that ensures that the population has sufficient income to enable it to eat and pay for a roof over its head, then health education which gives information about a 'healthy' lifestyle is unlikely to be very effective.

Thatcher and social security

The original consensus of 'Butskellite' (Rab Butler/Hugh Gaitskill) British politics of the 1950s and early 1960s over state welfare and welfare spending was already weakening to some extent in the late 1960s and the 1970s as concern grew over the increasing economic burden of welfare. This was exacerbated by economic problems caused by the oil crisis of 1973 and the resultant period of high inflation and growing unemployment in Britian. Nevertheless, though the Labour government of 1974–79 had presided over the earliest cuts in welfare spending it had remained firmly committed to the basic principles of the welfare state.

However Britain of 1979 bore little relation to that of 1947. In 1947 'there was a war warmed impulse for a more generous society' (Titmuss quoted by Krause in *The Guardian*, 1992). The principle of universal, state (i.e. public) welfare based on the idea of citizenship was embraced by all the political parties. Consensus was reached over support and maintenance of a comprehensive welfare state and policies of full employment and sustained economic growth.

In the ensuing 30 years changes in British society meant that social security provision had become extremely expensive to the tax payer. Demographic changes meant a large increase in the numbers of retirement pensioners; changes in marriage patterns meant there were many more single parents needing state benefit and the increasing numbers of unemployed people drawing benefit also had implications for the social security system.

By 1979 former wholehearted support for the Welfare State was being replaced by a less sympathetic approach to the poor and needy, fuelled by media exposures of 'scroungers'. The British people exhibited signs of lessening tolerance for others who needed state support. There was a general feeling amongst the electorate that certain people (the idlers) were getting something for nothing whilst they (the workers) were having to work hard to make ends meet in times of increasing economic hardship.

Thatcher's promise to roll back the frontiers of state, reduce taxes and restore the dynamism of the private sector found favour with the electorate, including many skilled working class voters who defected in droves from the Labour to the Conservative Party, thus giving the Conservatives a resounding majority in the Commons.

As an anticollectivist, Thatcher believes in minimal state intervention and in the value of inequality and individualism. In policy terms this means that welfare provision should be the responsibility of individuals and their families, not the state. Consequently 1979 saw the beginning of the development of policies which focus on the responsibility of the individual and/or the private sector to provide welfare support.

Thatcher inherited many problems in 1979 including high inflation and high unemployment. As a 'free marketeer' her main purpose has been to deal with high inflation by reducing interest rates and by privatizing nationalized industries, thus freeing the market to find its own level.

The problem of unemployment was not seen to be of particular importance; rather it was seen to be unfortunate but necessary – a market oriented economy has a low social commitment to full employment. Instead the emphasis is on 'lean' business enterprises working to full capacity for minimal costs, the key concepts being efficiency, economy and effectiveness. This, of course, is at odds with Beveridge who saw that full employment was essential to the welfare state.

In the years between 1946 and 1979 Beveridge's original principle of universality – minimum benefits available to all financed by a system of contribution rather than tax – had developed into a complex system of contributory and non-contributory benefits with additional benefits available to those who met specified criteria.

A feature of the social security system in 1979 had become the low uptake of benefit; a significant proportion of the available budget remained (and still remains) unspent each year because benefits were not claimed. There were many explanations for this phenomenon including, for example, the stigma attached to collecting benefit, the unhelpful attitude of some administrators, the difficulties of getting to the nearest social security office but above all the complexity of the benefit system itself.

As one way of overcoming this problem the social security system was simplified in 1988 under the Social Security Act (1986). One benefit that was retained was Child Allowance which had almost 100% uptake (child allowance is non-stigmatizing because every family with children is entitled to claim – it is not dependent on means testing). However this benefit has given rise to much political controversy. Thatcher was opposed on principle to universal benefits but was unable to persuade the Commons to abolish Child Allowance. Instead its value was effectively reduced by 'freezing' the amount paid for three successive years.

The Social Security Act (1986) introduced a new range of means tested benefits as follows:

Family Credit (replacing Family Income Supplement)

This is a benefit for working people who are employed or self-employed in fulltime low paid employment and have at least one child.

The amount of Family Credit that can be claimed is based on the number of children in the family and their ages, the income of the family including earnings and other social security benefits but excluding Child Benefit and Housing Benefit and the amount of savings that the family has.

Maximum payment is paid to families where net earned income is at or below the level of income support and will bring the income of that family above the level of income support. Thus families where one or more members are in fulltime employment are better off financially than those who are unemployed.

Family Credit entitles the recipients to NHS prescription charge exemption and other related exemptions.

Income Support (replacing Supplementary Benefit)

This is a state benefit for people whose income does not reach the government defined minimum for living (sometimes called the poverty line by analysts and academics (see Blackburn, 1991) but not by governments who do not officially acknowledge the term).

Income support can be 'topped up' by premiums – additional allowances for people with special needs. Examples include family premium, disability premium and pensioner premium and again the recipients are entitled to free NHS prescriptions and other related items including free school meals.

Free school meals are only available to the children of parents who are receiving Income Support, not those receiving Family Credit.

Housing Benefit

This is available where appropriate to help with the payment of rent and community charge/council tax.

Means tested benefits are only available to people with less than £6000 in savings and are reduced pro rata for people who have savings between £3000 and £6000.

Family Credit and Income Support are based on the premise that the determination of the overall financial entitlement of a household should be a straightforward predictable process resulting in a sum of money which is sufficient to live on but which will not remove incentive to work for those able to do so.

Means tested state benefits are available to those with insufficient finances to maintain a reasonable quality of life as defined by the state and so, in Beveridge's terms, act as a safety net. However, since Beveridge, dependence on means tested benefits has accelerated to the extent that the fiscal gap has widened inordinately. This has created enormous problems for a government which has pledged to reduce taxes.

Social Fund

The Social Fund is a scheme designed to help people on Family Credit or Income Support to meet exceptional expenses.

Grants, including a lump sum Maternity Needs Payment and a Death Grant to help with funeral expenses, are available and are means tested. Grants may also be available under the Social Fund to assist with the promotion of 'community care', especially in relation to people newly discharged from long-stay hospitals to live in the community. This grant could also be used to improve the living conditions of vulnerable or disadvantaged groups in the community.

A loan scheme, perhaps the most controversial element of the Social Fund, is in operation. This is intended to assist with the purchase of essential items such as furniture for people on Income Support.

The loan scheme is controversial on three counts. Firstly, though the loans are interest free they must be repaid and the repayment is deducted at source from the recipient's Income Support benefit so many people cannot afford the loan. Secondly, the central amount available for loans is cash limited so the money may run out before the end of the financial year. Bearing this in mind some social security officers have been parsimonious with the loans they have administered, especially at the beginning of the financial year. Thirdly, loans under the Social Fund are discretionary and require complex judgement. Though the DHSS officers administering the Fund are specially trained there have been anomalies in the loan system with major variations in the amount loaned and also in identification of what constitutes an appropriate loan.

Perhaps it is the Social Fund above all other changes in the social security system that demonstrates Thatcher's adherence to the ideology of the New Right. The Social Fund is an example of the minimal safety net allowed in a market economy; the state expects the family, charities and charitable institutions to fill the gap left by state provision.

One consequence of Thatcher's social security policies has been the development of a two-tier society in Britain, the haves and the have nots. Johnson (1990) states, 'The Conservatives have reversed the trends established in the 1970s of a narrowing of both income and wealth distribution' (p. 198) and 'Over the last 10 years the gap between benefits and wages has widened and the new social security system has served only to heighten the disparity' (p. 200).

Britain in 1994 has an increasing unemployment problem, a growing number of people who are homeless (officially classed as roofless) and a commensurate increase in the diseases of deprivation – tuberculosis and malnutrition.

The responsibility of the individual to provide for himself to meet the common hazards of life such as sickness, unemployment and old age has been exemplified in legislation and tax benefits in relation to occupational pensions and private health insurance. This has been productive for insurance companies but has left many with a feeling of unease and an increasing lack of confidence in the availability of state support should they need it.

CONCLUSION

It is probably too early to analyse the success or otherwise of Thatcher and post-Thatcher health and welfare policies in general – the success or failure may well depend on the perspective of the analyst! However, it is possible to offer an early evaluation in terms of how well the policies have addressed the problems that Thatcher inherited in 1979.

In 1994 accountability for the delivery of health care is easily traced. The observation, often attributed to Sir Roy Griffiths in 1982, that if Florence Nightingale were carrying her lamp through the corridors of the NHS today she would almost certainly be searching for the people in charge is no longer relevant.

Outcomes of health care are not only available but inform health care delivery. The NHS is still a bottomless pit into which resources could be thrown but resource management systems ensure that the resources are channelled effectively.

Money is now spent with more consideration and less waste, consequently more effectively and economically. Quality of care and customer satisfaction are the twin aims of every unit delivering health care and competition within the system ensures that these aims are met.

However, all is not well in many areas. There are mounting fears that quality is being sacrificed to economy as cost cutting exercises become more and more rigorous. Ward closures and job losses are becoming commonplace. Workforce and skill mix reviews have meant that highly qualified staff are fearful for their jobs – the morale amongst the staff is at rock bottom which must have an effect on the care they give.

The fundamental question that remains to be answered is how appropriate is a system of internal markets to a welfare state? Separating out the purchaser from the provider function has given a logic and consistency to health care delivery that was long overdue but can that logic extend to NHS trusts and GP fundholding practices? A market economy accepts that businesses rise and fall with the market and that some become casualties. However, is it appropriate that this should be applied to health care which is the fundamental right of everyone and should not have to depend on the success or failure of the local health 'business'? How long will the British citizen be able to retain the current level of confidence that if he is ill he will be able to obtain the best and most appropriate treatment free to him at the point of delivery? One task of the current and future governments is to provide answers to these questions.

The tasks of the current government in relation to social security are equally daunting, especially in times of a world recession and mounting unemployment.

Firstly a decision has to be made as to whether or not Britain can still afford a welfare state in the 1990s and if it can, how it will be financed. For example, should this be by increasing taxes or should the state subsidize premiums for private occupational pensions and health insurance? Or should the individual be left to fend for himself with the state offering only a minimal 'safety net' to those with no means of support, as is the current system in the USA?

One thing is certain: demographic changes and mounting unemployment mean that there are more and more people needing the safety net of the Welfare State and as the drain on the financial resources of the state increases, so taxation in some form must rise to meet this need.

We have already seen in this chapter how the British public became less altruistic about supporting the poor over the earlier years of the Welfare State, which eventually resulted in an election victory for the political party that promised to rationalize welfare state provision. Social policy has moved a long way from the original idealism of postwar Britain. Johnson (1990) states that Britain has become a more unequal society with more people living in poverty, a divided society in terms of occupation, housing, race and gender, rich and poor and a less democratic society. It remains to be seen whether the Welfare State will be dismantled altogether or, if it is to survive, how this will be achieved in the face of mounting odds and financial pressures.

REFERENCES

Blackburn, C. (1991) *Poverty and Health (Working with Families)*, Open University Press, Milton Keynes.

Cutler, T., Williams, K. and Williams, J. (1986) *Keynes, Beveridge and Beyond*, Routledge & Kegan Paul, London.

DHSS (1946) *The National Health Services Act*, HMSO, London.

DHSS (1972) *Report of the Committee on Nursing (Cmnd 5115)*, (The Briggs Report), HMSO, London.

DHSS (1973) *The National Health Services Reorganisation Act*, HMSO, London.

DHSS (1979) *Royal Commission on the National Health Service (Cmnd 76615)*, (The Merrison Report), HMSO, London.

DHSS (1983) *NHS Management Inquiry*, circular number DA (83)38, (The Griffiths Report), HMSO, London.

DHSS (1987) *Promoting Better Health*, HMSO, London.

DHSS (1990a) *Working for Patients*, HMSO, London.

DHSS (1990b) *The New GP Contract*, HMSO, London.

DHSS (1990c) *NHS & Community Care Act*, HMSO, London.

DoH (1991) *The Health of the Nation*, HMSO, London.

DoH (1992) *Health of the Nation: Strategy for Action*, HMSO, London.

Fraser, D. (1973) *The Evolution of the British Welfare State*, cited in Hill, M. (1988).

Ham, C. (1982) *Health Policy in Britain*, Macmillan, London.

Harrison, S. (1988) *Managing the National Health Service: Shifting the Frontier?*, Chapman & Hall, London.

Hill, M. (1988) *Understanding Social Policy*, 3rd edn, Blackwell, Oxford.

Johnson, N. (1990) *Reconstructing the Welfare State*, Harvester Wheatsheaf, New York.

Pierson, C. (1991) *Beyond the Welfare State*, Polity Press, Oxford.

Potter, D. (1982) *Politics, Legitimacy and the State – Unit 14, Open University D102, Block 4*, Open University Press, Milton Keynes.

Townsend, P. and Davidson, D. (eds) (1988) *Inequalities in Health (The Black Report and the Health Divide)*, Penguin, Harmondsworth.

Weale, A. (1983) *Political Theory and Social Policy*, Macmillan, London.

Wicks, M. (1987) *A Future for All: Do We Need a Welfare State?*, Penguin, Harmondsworth.

2

Lifestyle influences on client health

Monica Tettersell and Sarah Luft

Health is a product of society rather than nature or medicine.
(Hart, 1985)

INTRODUCTION

Health professionals, both in primary and secondary care, are increasingly involved with promoting the health of patients. Government legislation on health in recent years has done much to encourage a change of emphasis from a pure disease orientated system of health care to that which considers lifestyle and prevention of disease. This policy was initially identified in 1987 with the publication of the government White Paper entitled *Promoting Better Health* (DHSS, 1987). In the following year Sir Donald Acheson as Chief Medical Officer publicly stated that the government was convinced that shifting the balance of the National Health Service (NHS) in favour of disease prevention and health promotion was a vital key to improving the nation's health. The responsibilities for providing health promotion became explicit in 1989 in the NHS reforms *Working for Patients* produced by the Department of Health (1989) and more recently in the general practitioner contract introduced in April 1990 and the government White Paper *The Health of the Nation* (DoH, 1992).

The aim of these documents is to attempt to readjust the balance of the NHS from a 'disease service' to a 'health service' by expanding primary prevention activity. The main objective is to improve and increase health promotion activity, in particular in primary health care settings, in order to reduce premature morbidity and mortality. This change has been welcomed by most health professionals because the aim is commendable, although Klein (1983) would argue that the change in emphasis from medical engineering to social engineering has occurred only as a result of the incapability of medical science to produce health and the increasing health care expenditure. However, health promotion as interpreted by the reforms does not fit comfortably into a general practice setting, as it appears to overlook the influence that social phenomena have on health status.

It is widely accepted that preventive medicine is an integral component of good clinical practice and the promotion of positive health is not a new concept to primary health care. Prevention underpinned the National Health Services Act of 1946. This preceded the Peckham Experiment in the mid 1940s which reinforced the virtues of the activity (Pearce and Crocker, 1944). The Doctor's Charter pertaining to general practitioners, which was introduced in 1966, did much to lay the foundations for an increasing emphasis on prevention and health promotion in general practice (RCGP, 1981). By the late 1980s, prior to the introduction of the new general practitioner contract, interest in the field of health promotion and anticipatory care had increased significantly and extensive activity in this field was occurring.

DEFINING HEALTH

Most accepted definitions recognize that health does not purely mean being free from disease, although many lay people and some professionals may interpret it this way. Health is a complex and multifactorial issue influenced by the social, economic, cultural and physical environment in which people live. However, the recognition that health is a social phenomenon rather than a medical entity has led to an unrealistic utopia that health is 'a state of complete physical, mental and social well-being' (WHO, 1948). Health, rather like illness, means different things to different recognized people and this has to be accepted if one is engaged with the promotion of health.

Most lay people view the role of health professionals as assisting with 'sickness' or 'ill health'. It is assumed therefore that people visit a doctor's surgery when ill. The majority of health statistics on primary and secondary care are based on this assumption as they are compiled using consultation data. However, it would appear that a large percentage of ill health never reaches a doctor's surgery and various social factors influence an individual's decision to consult a professional or define themselves as being ill.

Epsom (1978) investigated the health status of 3160 adults, using a mobile health clinic; 57% of the cohort were referred to their general practitioner for further tests or treatment. This study demonstrates that people do not necessarily consult general practitioners for diseases that would respond to treatment.

It is a misconception that people who do not consult doctors are normally asymptomatic and symptoms do not lead people to define themselves as ill. Zola (1978) summarized several studies which demonstrated that apparently healthy people have symptoms of ill health on most days of their lives. Blaxter's (1976) study of middle aged Scottish women demonstrated that the women had developed and legitimized 'reasons' for ill health from their particular social setting. If it was possible to 'normalize' a symptom by a legitimized reason, they would not consult a doctor.

It is also important to consider what an individual's beliefs are on the perception of quality of life. An individual's personal evaluation of physiological, physical, psychological and social well-being may be perceived differently by the health professional.

People often seek the advice of family and friends about health matters rather than consult a professional. Helman (1978) suggested that lay or folk beliefs continue to survive the impact of modern medicine.

If unhealthy people are not consulting health professionals due to social phenomena, then to expect apparently 'healthy' people to consult for health promotion interventions could be viewed as naive. Alternative approaches for health promotion activity, such as community development, may best suit this group.

Primary care practitioners must accept that they have a central role to play in changing the lifestyles of individuals, families and populations (Smail, 1992). However, the assumption that medical and nursing professionals innately make ideal 'health educators' is misguided. Both professional groups have received education which encourages them to be essentially reactive to ill health, rather than proactive. Both are familiar with 'disease theory' and often naively believe that 'health' equates with 'absence of disease'. The result of this could be described as a 'Healthist approach' – 'health' being the ultimate value.

If, as it currently appears, health promotion is to continue in general practice, primary health care teams must examine their own values, beliefs and attitudes to the activity. Is it seen as worthwile? The medical profession has expressed concerns about the doubtful significance of health promotion interventions and indeed felt pressurized to accept their revised terms of service in April 1990 (GMSC, 1989). If this is true, then their scepticism may be reflected in the health messages they convey.

Industrialization in the nineteenth century brought about major improvements in sanitation and as a result eliminated many major infectious diseases. The public health problems, however, have been replaced with the so-called diseases of affluence, premature coronary heart disease, stroke and cancers. The concept of health and illness would appear to be a social rather than medical phenomenon.

SOCIAL CLASS

The effect of social class on health is well researched and there is extensive literature on the topic. For Black *et al.* (1990) social class is central to the development of work on inequality. They describe social class as segments of the population who share broadly similar types and styles of living and levels of resources, together with some sharing of perceptions. Bilton *et al.* (1992) refer to the crucial place of stratification in the organization of society and suggest that every aspect of the life of every individual and household is affected by stratification. Privileged groups are likely to enjoy certain basic forms of advantage, one of which is life chances. Bilton *et al.* maintain that these may include not only the economic advantages of wealth and income but also benefits such as health and job security. Based on theories of stratification these authors

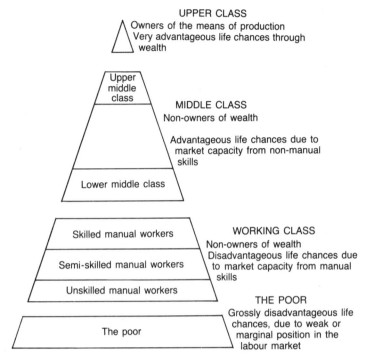

Figure 2.1 Marx and Weber three class model of contemporary capitalist society (reproduced with permission from Bilton *et al.*, 1992).

propose a three class model of contemporary capitalist societies; this model is outlined in Figure 2.1.

The Registrar General's Social Class Scale, used since 1911, is based on occupational grouping. Non-manual and manual refer to professional, intermediate, skilled, semi-skilled and unskilled manual groups. The semiskilled and unskilled manual workers comprise classes 4 and 5 and these occupations include agricultural workers, machine operators, telephone operators, barmen, bus conductors and railway porters among others. The literature shows that there are major differences in all aspects of health with a gradual deterioration from class I to class IV and a marked deterioration in social class V. People in the lowest two groups have higher standardized mortality ratios and increased levels of morbidity.

Theories which may explain some of the inequalities are proposed by Whitehead (1988). One of these postulates the culture/behavioural concept which incorporates the notion of responsibility in that the different social groups can choose their own particular lifestyles and that perhaps the lower socioeconomic groups have adopted behaviour patterns which are more dangerous and involve more health damaging behaviour than the higher socioeconomic groups. The other perspective proposes a materialist/structuralist explanation which places more blame on the environment because of the conditions under which some people work and live and the pressures on them to consume unhealthy products. According to Whitehead there is evidence to demonstrate that these two distinctions are interrelated rather than mutually exclusive. For instance, cigarette smoking supports such evidence in that there are figures available which demonstrate the prevalence of smoking in Great Britain both by sex and socioeconomic group, with the lower socioeconomic groups sharing a higher percentage of smokers.

Whitehead also refers to the differences in behaviour between the classes in relation to alcohol consumption, food and nutrition, and exercise in leisure time. However, although there is evidence which suggests that lifestyle itself can account for the differences in health between the classes it is certainly not the whole story and studies carrid out in the USA point strongly to the importance of an 'adequate' income. These studies suggest that behaviour patterns themselves are not the major factors in increased mortality, but that factors relating to the general living conditions and environment of the poor are more likely to be implicated. The materialist/structuralist theory which incorporates issues relating to housing and income does appear to demonstrate that adverse social conditions can limit the choice of lifestyle for an individual.

Chapman (1982) argues that there is evidence to show that the social class to which a person belongs may shape his life experience and affect his attitudes and values. This is reflected in family life, in the way children are reared and in the relationship which exists between husband and wife. There is also a connection between social class and education.

Historically the upper classes have enjoyed the benefits of further and higher education and despite the various education acts which have evolved over the years, there are inequalities and a relationship between social class and education still exists.

It is well documented that individuals from lower social classes find it more difficult to modify advice to fit their own perceived needs, since most advice is generally based on the values and beliefs of individuals from the middle and upper social classes. It is possible, for instance, that individuals who are 'socialized' within families where language deprivation exists and who are subsequently educated at schools which fail to instil further educational growth (because this is not valued at home) are disadvantaged when it comes to expressing their particular health care needs. The political emphasis currently reinforces the importance for health services to respond to the 'needs' of the population. Given a population where a high percentage are unable to articulate their needs, how can this be done? It seems that one of the fundamental problems here lies within the fabric of society itself in the reality of class differences which are integral to family life, to education and to the nature of the occupation undertaken by the individual.

Chapman cites Goldthorpe and Lockwood (1970) who documented comparisons between working class and middle class perspectives which categorize how they felt the different classes viewed the world around them. For instance they suggest that working class perspectives include the belief that 'What happens to you depends a lot on luck – otherwise you have to learn to put up with things'. The middle class view suggests that those who have the ability and initiative can overcome obstacles and create their own opportunities. Where someone ends up depends on what they make of themselves.

It is interesting to question whether these basic 'class' beliefs have changed over the past two decades. These beliefs for instance indicate a clear distinction between the two classes in that the middle class person takes responsibility for their life and actions while the working class individual supports the view that to a large extent they are victims of fate. To make clearcut generalizations today may be unwise as patterns of behaviour emerge which reflect current social norms. Unemployment in the 1990s has affected all classes – the middle classes, for instance, may now choose to describe themselves as 'victims of fate'.

It is worth mentioning that GPs are professionals who are classified in group 1 and their medical training has socialized them into a role which incorporates power. The working class individual in particular accepts such referent power and this attitude reinforces the notion of the 'social order' whereby the health professional has the authority and responsibility. The whole concept of general practice itself therefore may be perpetuating a 'them and us' scenario which is not conducive to self-responsibility.

POVERTY

In Victorian England many people regarded poverty as 'God given'; the individual concerned was responsible for their state because they were not helping themselves sufficiently. The concept of the Welfare State, however takes a different perspective in that it appears to recognize that the problem of poverty requires some form of collective social action. In recent years there has been ample evidence on how poverty can affect individual health status. The Black Report (1980) and later work by Whitehead (1988) reinforced this belief. Marmot and McDowell (1986) looked at death rates in men and women and concluded that although the overall mortality rates had fallen, the decline in manual workers was less than that of non-manual – in fact, the inequality had widened.

Bilton *et al.* refer to 'the culture of poverty' which proposes that poor people remain so because they have different values and ways of life from the rest of society. In other words they breed their own culture which in effect prevents them from achieving success or prosperity. Again, such a view tends to put the onus of responsibility for being poor back on to the individual, with the wider social and economic factors not being taken into consideration.

Poverty has been referred to as being 'relative', which means that a person is considered to be poor in relation to the accepted norms of society at the time. What is regarded as necessary for a decent standard of living is a matter of social definition and will change over time. Today, indoor amenities such as toilets and bathrooms and running hot water are regarded as necessities. If an individual's income falls markedly below those of other members in the community they may be considered poor, even if that income is adequate for survival. Poverty, therefore, needs to be considered in the light of the 'normal' material expectancies for society at a particular time. In the 1930s a person was thought to be affluent if he owned a vacuum cleaner. In the 1990s most people would expect to own such a utility.

There are certain categories of people who may be more vulnerable to poverty than others. These include the elderly, the disabled, the mentally ill, the large family, the single parent family, the unemployed and the insecurely employed low wage earner. These people may not be able to rely on a reasonable income to assist them towards maintaining healthy lifestyles and the health service on its own cannot make real inroads when such fundamental difficulties are present. The Black Report proposed that the improvement of health for poor disadvantaged groups required strong government measures. An increase in local authority spending on housing stock, for instance, would go some way toward eliminating the health divide which currently exists.

ETHNICITY

It is known that members of ethnic minorities are over-represented in the lower socioeconomic classes and so they share many of the same problems as others in that particular group. Bilton *et al.* point out that many coloured immigrants have been recruited to fill lower working class occupational positions and hence suffer the low status, material and environmental disadvantages experienced by many white manual workers. This chapter acknowledges that health is linked to various kinds of poverty: low income, poor diet, unemployment, poor housing, large families, detrimental work conditions, polluted environments and inadequate access to health care are some of the factors which play a major role in determining the health of minority groups.

Many immigrants arrived in the United Kingdom during the 1950s and 1960s with large numbers settling within inner city areas where employment was available. These inner city areas have witnessed a marked decline over the last two decades with regard to industry and resources generally. This has led to an 'out migration' for many people but there exists still a significant number of people from different ethnic backgrounds who are living within inner cities in accommodation which is recognized as being substandard. As a consequence of linguistic and cultural differences, certain sections of the community may be excluded from health promotion activities. For example, the social/cultural characteristics of Asian women suggest that they may be more reluctant to seek professional medical help. This may be due to the attitudes towards health that are held within their own communities as well as the general practice of seeking help from informal sources. There may also be concern that there could be cultural misunderstanding and a possibility of a mismatch of values between themselves and the health professionals.

Storkey (1991) points to the figures relating to the infant mortality rates in the UK. In 1961 the UK had a lower infant mortality rate than any country in the European community other than Denmark and the Netherlands, but in 1985 it had a higher rate than anywhere other than Greece, Italy and Portugal. These figures are startling given the advances in medical technology that have occurred over the years. More specifically, a study of normal pregnancies delivered in 1980 indicated that 11.3% of Indian babies and 10% of Pakistan babies were classified as being of lower birth weight compared with 7.3% of European babies. The figure for West Indian babies was close to the Pakistan figure. Storkey refers to a report from the Community Relations Commission in 1977 which revealed further information and provides a clearer picture. These include greater incidences of:

- iron deficiency and pernicious anaemia
- rickets
- sickle cell disease
- jaundice
- ulcers.

More recently attention has focused on studies which indicate a higher level of cancer amongst those of African origin.

These disturbing figures demonstrate the need to target health promoting activities for ethnic groups. According to Storkey, these women are among the lowest paid in the country and British West Indian women form a significant proportion of single parents. Discrimination with regard to race can be viewed in the same way as those in poverty. There tends to be a self-perpetuating process which prevents these groups from improving their situation and one must seriously question whether people from different ethnic backgrounds have equal opportunities which would enable them to acquire improved life chances. Do they in fact receive the opportunities to obtain the appropriate skills and qualifications which would enable empowerment? The Community Relations Commission cited research which suggested, for instance, that Asians who spoke little English were in low status, low paid jobs living within an extended family in poor quality accommodation for which they had to pay high rents or mortgages.

Many of these points are supported by Hart 1985 who stresses that it is not the individual who is to blame for engaging in 'unhealthy' behaviours but the current system of cultural beliefs which fail to reach certain sections of society. There is evidence to suggest that the majority of the literature currently published to reinforce health education messages is aimed at the white middle classes, not the groups who may be in most need.

LIFE EVENTS

Life events have been referred to as 'normative' in that they are those events that are likely to affect all of us at some time in our lives – examples include changing schools, getting married, having children and retiring. Some life events which occur for many people but which are not considered the norm are referred to as 'idiosyncratic' and examples of these may be divorce, death of a child or a major illness. The normative life events are to a large extent expected and people adapt and make the required changes in their lives in order to cope with the event.

Niven (1989) identifies two approaches within primary prevention which may alleviate some of the associated stress connected with life events. There is a need firstly to consider the prediction and understanding of physical and pyschological disorder in a population as a function of its association with life events and secondly to consider the process by which life events facilitate adaption, development and 'growth' in an individual.

There is a lot of research that indicates that life events have a strong influence on the health status of an individual. Brown's study (1986) of 395 working class mothers in Islington considered the relationship between life events, internal resources, social support and onset of depression. Low self-esteem and poor social support increased vulnerability to developing depression and ill health.

Welin *et al.*'s longitudinal study of Swedish civil servants and coronary heart disease risk also demonstrated that social support was a crucial influencing factor to health status.

When individuals recognize an unhealthy behaviour in themselves, they can often produce an internal rationale or personal justification for the activity. From their point of view they need to consider if it is in their best interests to deny themselves pleasurable activities, which are often props to social problems. As Smail (1992) states, 'Many people do not believe that basic self-care practices are relevant to their health and fail to understand how changes in practices could improve their health'. The degree to which individuals are permitted to determine interventions to their lifestyle requires attention, otherwise skilled efforts will be in vain.

Traditional folk beliefs about health will affect health interventions. What health professionals may view as important and worthwhile life changes may be dismissed by the individual.

Many people see health as the responsibilty of 'local councils' as they view it in social terms rather than as an exclusively medical preserve. If health problems are tackled without the underlying social problems, then health professionals will only be covering up the real cause. External factors and the roles they play in the generation of ill health must be acknowledged instead of placing the sole responsibility on the client.

In practice, it has to be asked who is attracted to attend health check-ups in general practice? Mainly 'the worried well'; most surgeries are inundated by them, representing a trend hat health promotion is becoming a comforter for the middle classes. Many of those attending only do so because they are aware that their lifestyles and social economic position allow them to live a reasonably healthy lifestyle. Is the activity only serving to meet the needs of a social elite? How many obese, heavy alcohol consuming, heavy smokers are seen queuing up outside a health promotion clinic to be reprimanded by a well meaning nurse about activities which they feel unable to control? Yet research confirms that these are the people who are at greatest risk from premature death. Tudor Hart (1971) described an inverse care law related to health provision and the economy and this is reflected in health promotion activity. Statistics from the OPCS (1978) and Blaxter (1976) show that the use of some preventative services increases as one moves up the social hierarchy.

Users and providers of health promotion activities need to understand each other's expectations. What does the patient want to achieve and, more realistically, what can they expect to achieve in their social setting? The work of health promotion clinics tends to be defined by the providers rather than the users. It is essential that activity is centred around the individual and not the health professional.

WHAT IS HEALTH PROMOTION?

The World Health Organization describes health promotion as, 'The process of enabling people to increase control over and improve their health' (1948). In recent years the terms health promotion and health education have been interchanged so consistently that the words appear synonymous. This is, however, far from the true definitions which are distinctly different activities. Health promotion can be defined as a process which considers personal and cultural experience within the social, economic and environmental circumstances. Health education is aimed at encouraging voluntary behaviour changes and does not include organizational economic and environmental support.

The government's expectations from the health promotion process in general practice appear to be over ambitious. When the true meaning of health promotion is considered, general practice can realistically only offer health education and is less likely to be able to involve a multidimensional approach. Should health promotion be centred in general practice, as this approach encourages a myopic view of addressing health? It predominantly identifies medical health needs and frequently overlooks social needs.

The medical profession, accepting the responsibility for health promotion, will continue to fight an insurmountable task, if viewed in isolation. Current NHS prevention activity is well described by Irving Zola's (1978) river analogy in that, 'What health professionals seem to be doing is pulling people out of the river and attempting to resuscitate them, rather than looking up the river and finding out who's pushing them in'.

Unless primary health care workers engage the realities of poverty, then their impact on health will be limited and fundamental health problems will continue (Becker, 1990). General practitioners and nursing staff must be prepared to become involved with public health issues if they seriously hope to have any significant impact on the health of their practice population. Emphasis on target setting and process audit creates a conveyer belt approach to health promotion which will result in little or no health gain.

Government policy would appear to place the responsibility for an individual's health in two camps. On one hand the medical profession (general practitioners in particular) have a duty to undertake this activity under their contractual terms of service and as a result have become an 'agency' responsible for promoting health. On the other hand, individuals are expected to permit professionals to 'health promote' them, to become passive recipients of health advice and as a result, assume more responsibility for their health, changing behaviours which are judged to be detrimental to health.

The government White Paper *The Health of the Nation* (DoH, 1992) and the GP Contract (DHSS, 1990) and revised contract (DoH, 1993) concentrate predominantly on coronary heart disease prevention as this continues to be a major cause of premature death in the UK. The target set by the government is to reduce coronary heart disease by 30% by the year 2000 (DoH, 1992). The encouraged activity would appear to land health care professionals with the moral responsibility for the unacceptable high levels of morbidity and mortality from coronary heart disease. However, the fundamental problems of inequality of health status fail to be addressed by the proposed strategies. The White Paper is modelled on the World Health Organization strategy for health by the year 2000, which produces broader targets aimed at reducing existing inequities in health. Sadly, unlike its precursor, the White Paper fails to recognize that health promotion must be viewed in a social and economic context.

It is inaccurate to believe that health promotion can be described in terms of an activity – 'Is it possible to "health promote" someone?' Surely the promotion of health is not an activity but an aspiration. The World Health Organization declaration at Alma Ata in 1978 (WHO, 1978) stated that health is a fundamental right of every human being.

McKeown (1979) believes that the main determinants of health are external and there is much evidence to suggest he is right in this. However, a purist lifestyle approach to health promotion based on targets is inappropriate and places stress on individuals and encourages victim blaming. Nutbeam (1986) describes victim blaming as the belief that an individual has the chief responsibility for their health, which neglects the infuence of the social, economic and physical environment and the constraints on lifestyles imposed by these factors. Patients are labelled as deviant or non-compliant if they do not conform as expected.

People are reluctant or refuse to heed advice for many reasons, which warrant further discussion. Current health promotion activity in general practice leans too heavily on expecting individuals to change their lifestyles and does not consider how this can be achieved. Attempts to alter people's behaviour must be linked with an individual's psychosocial factors and health beliefs. Health promotion does not mean telling people how to behave, persuading or manipulating them, controlling and coercing, often against their will, in the naive belief that they will alter their behaviour. It is about respecting the autonomy of the individual and empowering them to make healthy life choices.

The influence that social circumstances have on health status is seemingly ignored in the White Paper *The Health of The Nation*. This represents a naivety in government circles, which in turn questions the content (George, 1992); Cole-Hamilton, 1991). General practice must not be viewed as the only setting where intervention occurs otherwise health is in danger of becoming 'medicalized'.

Heath intervention activity in general practice can only be viewed as one facet in a national programme. It is essential that other agencies are involved in raising public awareness of health issues and empowering them to adopt healthier lifestyles. Local strategies based on need must be collaboratively set if as a nation we are to tackle the fundamental problems affecting the health of the nation which include poverty, poor housing, low incomes and environmental problems.

The WHO strategy 'Health for All 2000' advocates a community development approach to promoting health in which people have a right and duty to participate individually and collectively in the planning and implementation of health care. People in a community are helped to define their needs and to negotiate how these should be met in collaboration with those who control the resources. Benefits include:

- An opportunity to readdress inequalities by acting on underlying social and economic determinants of health.
- Giving consideration to both individuals and their local community's perceptions of need which are frequently very different to government and medical definitions. Lay people see health as problems embedded within the social and economic fabric of life. There is very little point talking to people about lowering their daily fat consumption, eating brown bread and jogging if their fundamental problems are associated with social and economic deprivation.
- Allowing the community to participate in policy planning and development of services which they identify are needed. So the community defines its own health needs, thus breaking away from a top-down approach to defining need.
- Encouraging collaboration between health services and other statutory and voluntary agencies, to develop a comprehensive and integrated strategy.
- Avoiding victim blaming.

A difficulty that most practices have about this approach is the definition of a 'community'. In theory the idea of this being a geographical locality is laudable, but most practice teams would see it in terms of the practice population. This argument is academic as the approach is clearly the same but on a larger population.

Increasingly nurses are involved with anticipatory and preventive care in the general practice setting. This has mainly occurred because general practitioners do not view the activity as an integral part of their role and also because of other service demands put on them. The number of nurses employed by general practitioners has risen dramatically since the mid 1980s as a result of increased activity in this area (Tettersell *et al.*, 1992). Research has demonstrated that nurses involved in organized health promotion activity can have better results than usual care offered by general practitioners (Drury *et al.*, 1987).

Nurses involved with health promotion need training to develop their role. This training should not only focus on the physiological effects of lifestyle on health but on the broader subject areas such as the social influences and how to encourage behavioural changes. Education should promote multidisciplinary interventions including colleagues from health and social services. No sole individual can be accountable for the health of the practice population.

Local interventions must be multiprofessional and involve other agencies such as social service departments, housing departments, education authorities, as well as voluntary agencies and the patients themselves. A practice nurse could be viewed as the co-ordinator for these agencies.

If general practice premises are to be a central focus for health promotion activity, they should reflect a healthy message. Thought and planning must be given to producing notice boards which convey health promotional advice. Researchers have demonstrated that only the minority read messages on notice boards, so it should not be the only medium for communication to patients. It may be more effective to place posters in other public places in the community, such as libraries, community centres, schools and workplaces, which establish a theme.

Relevant back-up material such as leaflets and audio-visual aids are useful additions. These need to be relevant for all social classes and reflect different cultural beliefs. Leaflets produced by the primary health care team for their own patients which reflect local needs may be most effective.

Health activities must be accessible to patients, so consideration has to be given to the timing and venue of activity. A casualty of the general practitioner contract of 1990 was opportunistic screening and anticipatory care, as general practitioners were encouraged to adopt a clinic approach. Fowler and Gray (1983) estimated that over 70% of the patients on a general practitioner's list will consult at least once in any given year and when extended to any member of the primary health care team, this equates to 90%. Over a five year period a general practitioner will see approximately 95% of registered patients. If patient contacts are capitalized, then opportunistic screening and interventions can be far reaching. The patient's motivation for intervention at the time of ill health may also be enhanced.

Primary health care teams need to collaborate on improving the health of the communities they serve, so an intersectoral approach should be fostered. This is frequently difficult as individual practitioners are inundated with individual patients' problems and rarely have an opportunity to stand back and view holistically the health needs of the community. However, an assessment of needs based on the health status of the population must be conducted if an intervention programme is to be effective.

The needs will vary upon the location of the practice and the population it serves. Following an assessment, local 'health targets' can be identified and priorities set for intervention. Most practices will have a mixture of client groups with different needs so the intervention activities must reflect this diversity.

CONCLUSION

This chapter opened by stating the government's intention of creating a health service rather than a disease service. Klein (1983) has reservations about what this means and the difficulties in achieving it: 'If the aim of the NHS is to eradicate disease and disability, it is self-evidently a failure. If, however, its role is defined as being to minimize human suffering, then it can be reckoned as a reasonable success story'.

Nurses and other health professionals engaged in general practice are in a pivotal position to contribute to health strategies, but they cannot be solely responsible. The contribution of social and economic disadvantages to ill health must be tackled otherwise any improvements to the health of the nation will be marginal. It is also essential that different cultural attitudes and beliefs are given serious consideration, otherwise inequality in certain sections of the community will be reinforced. People may appear biologically similar but it is different experiences, life expectations and social outlooks which make them individual.

A lifestyle approach cannot be the totality of health promotional activity as many causes of ill health are outside the influence of the individual. Those who require most help to improve their health are the least likely to attend health promotion clinics – thus the health divide expands.

Although primary health care workers can widen their vision and approach to health promotion, they cannot work in isolation. One must inevitably question the mortality of a government that continues to overlook the influence of economic and social factors on health.

REFERENCES

Acheson, D. (1988) *Public Health in England: The Report of the Committee of Inquiry into the Future Development of Public Health Function*, HMSO, London.

Becker, S. (1990) The sting in the tail. *Community Care*, April 12 1990; 22–4.

Bilton, T., Bonnett, K., Jones, P., Sandworth, M., Sheard, K. and Webster, A. (1992) *Introductory Sociology*, 2nd edn, Macmillan, Basingstoke.

Black, D. (1980) Inequalities in health. Report of a research working group chaired by Sir Douglas Black in, *Inequalities in Health*, (eds. P. Townsend and N. Davidson), Penguin, Harmondsworth.

Black, D., Morris, J. N., Smith, C., Townsend, P. and Whitehead, M. (1990) Inequalities in health, in *Society and Social Science: A Reader*, (eds J. Anderson and M. Ricci), Open University Press, Milton Keynes.

Blaxter, M. (1976) Social class and health inequalities, in *Equalities and Inequalities in Health*, (eds C. Carter and J. Peel), Academic Press, London.

Brown, G. (1986) Depression: a sociological view, in *Basic Readings in Medical Sociology*, (eds D. Tuckett and J. Kaufert), Tavistock Press, London.

Chapman, C. (1982) *Sociology for Nurses*, 3rd edn, Baillière Tindall, London.

Cole-Hamilton, I. (1991) Poverty makes you sick. *Poverty*, **80**, 12–15.

DHSS (1987) *Promoting Better Health*, HMSO, London.

DHSS (1989) *Working for Patients*, HMSO, London.

DHSS (1990) *General Practice in the National Health Service. A New Contract*, HMSO, London.

DoH (1992) *The Health of the Nation*, HMSO, London.

DoH (1993) *GP Contract Health Promotion Package*, NHS Management Executive SHS1 (93 3), HMSO, London.

Drury, M., Greenfield, S., Stillwell, B. and Hull, F. (1987) A nurse practitioner in general practice: patient perceptions and expectations. *Journal of the Royal College of General Practitioners*, **38**, 503–5.

Epsom, J. (1978) The mobile health clinic: a report on the first year's work, in *Basic Readings in Medical Sociology*, (eds D. Tuckett and J. Kaufert) Tavistock Press, London.

Fowler, G. and Gray, M. (1983) Opportunities for prevention in general practice, in *Preventive Medicine in General Practice*, (eds M.J. Gray and G. Fowler), Oxford University Press, Oxford.

General Medical Services Committee (1989) Report to a special conference of representatives of local medical committees, 27 April, British Medical Association, London.

George, M. (1992) The missing links. *Nursing Standard*, **6** (52), 20–1.

Hart, N. (1985) *Sociology of Health and Medicine*, Causeway Press, Ormskirk.

Helman, C. (1978) Feed a cold, starve a fever. *Culture Medicine and Psychiatry*, **2**, 107–37.

Klein, R. (1983) *The Politics of the National Health Service*, Longman, London.

Marmot, M. and McDowell, M. (1986) Mortality decline and widening social inequalities. *Lancet*, **2**, 274–6.

McKeown, T. (1979) *The role of Medicine: Dream, Mirage or Nemesis?* Blackwell, Oxford.

Niven, N. (1989) *Health Psychology: An Introduction for Nurses and Other Health Care Professionals*, Churchill Livingstone, Edinburgh.

Nutbeam, D. (1986) Health promotion glossary. *Health Promotion*, **1** (1), 113–27.

Office of Population Censuses and Surveys (1978) *Occupational Mortality Decennial Supplement 1970–72*, HMSO, London.

Pearce, A. and Crocker, L. (1944) *The Peckham Experiment: A Study in the Living Structure of Society*, George Allen & Unwin, London.

Royal College of General Practitioners (1981) *Health and Prevention in Primary Care*, Royal College of General Practitioners, London.

Smail, S. (1992) Health promotion and primary care, in *Screening and Surveillance in General Practice* (eds C. Hart and P. Burke), Churchill Livingstone, London.

Storkey, E. (1991) *Block 2 Social Structures and Divisions Unit 8 Race Ethnicity and Gender*, The Open University, Milton Keynes.

Tettersell, M., Sawyer, J. and Salisbury, C. (1992) *Handbook for Practice Nursing*, Churchill Livingstone, London.

Tudor Hart, J. (1971) The inverse care law. *Lancet*, 1, 405–12.

Welin, L., Tibblin, G., Svardsudd, K., Ander-Perciva, S., Larsson, B. and Wilhelmsen, L. (1985) Prospective study of social influences on mortality. *Lancet*, 1, 915–18.

Whitehead, M. (1988) The health divide, in *Inequalities in Health*, (eds P. Townsend and N. Davidson), Penguin, Harmondsworth.

World Health Organization (1948) *Health Promotion – A Discussion Document on the Concepts and Principles*, WHO, Copenhgen.

World Health Organization (1978) *Report of the International Conference on Primary Health Care*, Alma-Ata, USSR, 6–12 September, Health for All series No. 1, WHO, Geneva.

Zola, I. (1978) Pathways to the doctor, in *Basic Readings in Medical Sociology*, (eds D. Tuckett and J. Kaufert), Tavistock Press, London.

3

Managing health care in general practice

Alison Allcock

INTRODUCTION

The publication of the Patients' Charter (1992) has brought about a whole new approach to community and hospital care. Gone is the idea that the health service is in charge of the patient. Patients' rights are now at the forefront. They have the right to demand a service that reaches a set standard.

Good management within this healthcare system is needed now more than ever before. Cuts in resources mean that more efficient and effective ways have to be continually found to meet these preset standards. An essential element for the achievement of this is effective teamwork, from all health care specialties concerned. Basic management techniques such as teamwork, communication skills and motivation theory, that have been used in private industry for years, are now being incorporated into the health service. General practice is no exception. It has to be managed so that it is able to provide a service that is acceptable, accessible and able to meet the needs of the population it seeks to serve.

THE STRUCTURE OF THE ORGANIZATION

Practice nurses are becoming more involved than ever before in managing both patient care and the system in which they work. In any organization the efficiency with which the product or service is produced reflects the management skills behind its operation. If practice nurses can understand

and use the basic concepts of organizational structure and management then they too can offer an efficient service.

There are a variety of factors which interrelate within any organization, influencing its effectiveness. Studying some of these variables helps to highlight the complexity of management. Organization theory can be applied to experiences and functions within the practice and aid understanding about how these variables affect work, the aim being that in order to change a system for the better it is necessary first of all to understand the system. Throughout this chapter management theory that is often applied to industry will be related to general practice. Some aspects of the theory may seem removed from day-to-day patient consultation but on reflection this is far from true. The organization behind these consultations, for example, may be the key to their success.

A patient now has access to both medical and nursing services on first contact with a general practice. Nursing services may range from the diagnosis and treatment of acute and chronic illnesses to health promotion and screening services. Chronic diseases such as asthma and diabetes are now often dealt with in the practice setting by the practice nurse rather than in hospital. The co-ordination of these services necessitates a management structure. The members of a team are sometimes unaware of the existence of such a structure, but close examination will always reveal its presence.

The introduction of health promotion clinics into general practice has faced nurses with the task of managing their own activities. In a hospital, a nurse carrying out a procedure will always have an immediate superior giving instructions; for example, a staff nurse will have a sister, a sister her nurse manager. In general practice this type of hierarchy simply does not exist. The larger practices may have a senior nurse responsible for several others, but many of these will have their own specialty and may be the responsible nurse for a specific form of care. For example, such practices may well have their own specialized asthma nurse, diabetes nurse and family planning nurse, each of whom should have attended recognized training courses in their field. They are unlikely to have received structured training in organizational management and will therefore often be placed in situations where they have to use their own initiative and common sense. Such qualities are particularly valuable and this is shown by the success of the many nurse-run health promotion clinics up and down the country. The example of setting up a health promotion clinic will be used to highlight management theory. However, before that it is important to understand the organization to which this management theory is to be applied.

Figure 3.1, taken from Handy (1988) is an illustration of the complexity of variable factors associated with the effectiveness of an organization. The organization we are talking about is general practice but the same principles are applied to any organization although factors mentioned will vary from

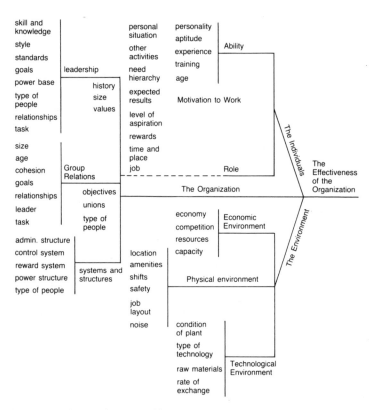

Figure 3.1 Some factors affecting organization effectiveness (reproduced with permission from Handy, 1988).

one practice to another. There are certain key areas that can be pulled from the diagram which are known to have an effect on an organization. For example, leadership styles will vary depending on the individuals in the leadership posts. Individuals involved at all levels within the organization will also affect the motivation factor and hence it can be seen why leadership and motivation are linked together.

The lower half of the diagram shows factors that are linked to the environment within which the work is taking place.

The important factors that affect an organization will be discussed later but to prove that nurses already know the basics behind management concepts, the first issue to be examined will be one that is familiar: the setting up of a health promotion clinic.

THE MANAGEMENT OF HEALTH PROMOTION

The concept of health promotion is now recognized as vital in general practice and so makes great calls upon the skills of the practice nurse and the primary health care team. This chapter does not define how to set up a clinic, it seeks to highlight the mechanisms and theoretical concepts behind the organization. The four steps defined by McKinsey (cited by Pritchard 1981), listed below, are essential for any successful organizational development and the implementation of change:

- Planning stage
- Motivation
- Initiation
- Evaluation.

These four stages are briefly examined in relation to their application to the health promotion clinic. They are then examined in more depth as issues in management.

The planning stage

Here the objectives are marked out and the method used to achieve these objectives is decided.

The planning stage of a health promotion clinic would involve the following:

- Identify the aim of the clinic
- Identify the target group
- Decide how the target group is to be reached
- Decide what the intended outcomes for the group are
- Recruit personnel to run the clinic
- Assess the length of time needed before evaluation is to be effective
- Devise a protocol that implements the above objectives and outcomes. A protocol serves as a guide for all team members and ensures that there is no conflict of input to a given area. Everyone should therefore work to the same guidelines to achieve an agreed objective. A protocol can be used to define a specific procedure, for example how to take a blood pressure, so that all members act in a consistent way or it can be more generalized. It is not possible to write standard protocols which are acceptable to every practice. Each protocol should be tailormade to fit the activity it sets out to standardize.

Once the protocol has been agreed the chain of events leads onto the next phase.

Motivation

This is the first stage of implementing the plan before its actual initiation. Motivation requires an agreement from all parties on the shared goals and enthusiasm for their achievement.

In the example of setting up a clinic it may well be that staff who are expected to work in the clinic have to be trained to carry out procedures required of them. This includes reception, administration, medical and nursing staff. A nurse relies on the administration team to work with her to achieve an efficient and well run clinic. Details such as booking systems, clinic location and equipment required would be discussed at this stage and any necessary purchases made. The date of commencement is important. There should be an agreed date for the start of the clinic which benefits both staff and patients alike.

Staff can be motivated by including them in the planning stage. They will then be able to identify with their roles at an early stage and understand the importance of them.

The motivation stage is a period of time that allows for preparation and for any likely problems to be teased out. If this stage is missed out, it can affect the long term success of the clinic. Motivation also requires sustaining once the initial enthusiasm wanes: this can be difficult to achieve and often tests the ingenuity of the team leader.

Initiation

The plan is put into action. This should be one of the easiest phases if the two prior ones have been explored to the full.

The clinic would proceed as per protocol devised in the planning stage. A set time for this phase should have been agreed before the clinic is to be evaluated. An average time for this stage would be three months which would allow for early problems to be ironed out.

Evaluation

The final stage before the process starts again. All nurses are now familiar with this term which is a sign that nursing is becoming more management based in its action. Evaluation and audit are terms commonly used by the practice nurse. It is at this stage that questions are answered:

- Have the functions and objectives of the protocol been reached?
- Is the uptake of the clinic a success?
- Has the protocol been followed or do parts of it need to be changed to conform with what is already happening?
- What else needs changing?

Figures can be used to monitor the success, i.e. attendance can be monitored.

Evaluation should be a continuous process, but its success depends on the action taken because of it. There is no sense in auditing if no change takes place after the event. Any problems perceived should be examined with a view to solving them rather than merely being aware of them.

These four stages soon become a circle of events. When problems are highlighted in the evaluation phase, it is necessary to return to the planning stage to solve them.

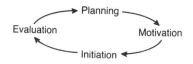

Figure 3.2 The circle of events for successful change.

By describing the four steps followed to set up a clinic, it becomes clear how health care workers do follow basic management techniques without perhaps being aware of it. This is true for other areas of management and having explained the basic principles, more specific areas can now be discussed.

THE MANAGEMENT OF CHANGE

One of the problems of general practice, or in fact any system that requires planning and management, is that there is constant change within the system. This is very much in evidence at the moment. No sooner have many systems been implemented than the government changes the policies. A good example of this is health promotion clinics. This is where evaluation is essential. Before changing any system there has to be some measure of its effectiveness before change can be warranted. Although change may be imposed on some aspects, it should not mean that what is successful needs to be changed as well. This is seen in the government's attitude towards health promotion and the new banding system. Clinics that are already up and running need not be changed if their original objective for being set up is being met.

Change is often inevitable in any line of trade, especially in the present economic climate. Some people view change with enthusiasm while others may feel threatened. This may have something to do with who is initiating the change. Research has shown that people who are most active in organizing any change seem to get the most benefits from it (Open University, 1988c).

This is simple to understand if related to our own situation. By simply thinking of some recent changes that have occurred at work and then answering the simple questions listed below, the sort of change that is easiest to cope with can be established. Think of two changes that you have been involved with, one that appeared easy and one that seemed more problematical:

- Was the change imposed?
- Who initiated it?
- Was it resisted?'
- Was it easy to cope with?
- Was it useful in its effects?
- Was it an effective change in your circumstances?

It would be expected that the changes that you have initiated are the most useful and easiest to cope with. In good management, change can be introduced more easily by making everyone concerned feel they are part of the planning and initiation.

What is change?

Kurt Lewin, a psychologist, originally described the simplest and most useful method for establishing the need for change in his force-field analysis (Lewin, 1951). This explains how, in any situation where there is equilibrium, there are two sets of forces working against each other to create the balance. These two forces are known as restraining forces and driving forces. When these are equal any situation remains static.

Let us return to the initial model of starting up a health promotion clinic to establish some of its driving and restraining forces (see Figure 3.3). This example illustrates that every situation, whether in industry or outside, has forces driving it to change and forces restraining it.

In order for change to occur the driving forces have to be stronger than the restraining forces and this can be promoted by either creating more driving forces or by reducing the restraining forces. It is worth noting at this stage that the forces will vary depending on who is analysing or devising the list. Often the majority of restraining forces exist because of the attitudes of people involved. For example, the necessity for staff to be trained could be a driving force rather than a restraining force if all staff wanted to be trained. The most sensible step when planning change is to list the variety of forces. This list should be drawn up by the team of people who will be

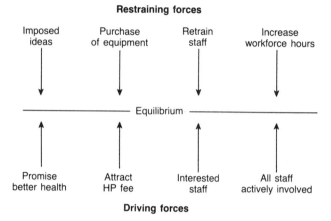

Figure 3.3 Examples of restraining and driving forces.

involved in any consequent change. Returning once again to the original plan, we can now see how important the planning stage is in any management work.

How should change best be managed if it is to be more acceptable to the people it affects? The fact that change imposed on people is less easily accepted than when it is initiated from within has already been discussed. It is for this reason that there is always resistance to government plans when change is imposed in the health care sector. Essentially if people are always prepared for and expect change even when no specific changes are imminent, it becomes easier to accept.

For this reason there is a constant need to be alert to the possibility of change in the environment in which people work. Change will then not be so difficult to accept when it happens. In an ideal world change should only be implemented if it is to achieve some specific improvement in the quality of service provided. Sadly in today's climate, change is often instigated as a cost cutting exercise rather than to accomplish this desired improvement. Even when imposed, the driving and restraining forces should be highlighted at the earliest stage by all who are concerned. This allows for the essential period of preparation, or motivation as it is classed in McKinsey's management structure, so that any possible problems can be aired before the initiation of the programme takes place.

Even though change may be imposed it is still essential that a record of cost is kept. This should be the cost of time, effort, resources, etc. so that evaluation becomes an easier process.

How can resistance to change be overcome?

When first introduced, the practice profiles and annual practice reports seemed a waste of time to many GPs. However they did make practices take a step back and look at the services they provided and then identify loopholes and gaps that could be further developed.

Sadly, however, the necessity for change often brought about by these reports can be disabled by many practice members. Opponents to change must be convinced of the reasons and advantages if it is going to be effective.

In order for resistance to be overcome it is essential that the people who will be ultimately affected are identified. The reasons why they may be resistant to the change should be highlighted and a problem solving approach could be employed to reduce the amount of resistance. Resisters should be given the chance to contribute to the change by suggesting modifications, and willingness should be shown so that justifiable modifications are taken on board and used.

Practice meetings are essential in such circumstances. They serve to keep all parties up to date on current issues and gain necessary support from key members for any projects underway.

Any results the change may bring about for these individuals can be discussed at this point. Honesty is essential so that grudges are spoken about and not harboured. However, it is important that emotional opposition is converted into constructive suggestions, otherwise there will be no headway.

This sort of thinking can also be adapted to patient care. Patient compliance is far more successful when the patient has had a say in the treatment decision. A nurse should always be aware of any resistance to ideas by the patient and adopt a similar approach to that which is used in the management of change.

TEAMWORK AND LEADERSHIP

Nursing in general practice was originally thought of as an isolated role. Many nurses found the change from busy hospital life to the relative solitude of a GP practice difficult to cope with. The nursing hierarchy had been removed along with nursing colleagues. Some doctors, however, have long been used to working in this isolation, singlehanded practices being quite the norm within the history of general practice and the idea of working as part of a team seemed quite foreign.

A team approach offers definite advantages, Handy (1988) suggests. Teamwork in general practice has evolved due to the number of health care specialists now working in the community. This group of professionals with a variety of skills now come together to work, one hopes, with the same objectives as each other, thus creating the primary health care team, which will be used as an example of teamwork.

The size of the team matters – a team is as large as the number of people who work within it to help achieve the agreed goal. This may sound obvious but sometimes crucial members are forgotten. For example, a doctor's receptionist is a vital member and although not offering hands-on advice or treatment to a patient, the team would soon break down without this input. Therefore, for any team to function effectively, individual members must be aware of all other members and value their role.

When studying the individuals often associated with or included in the primary health care team, one is struck by the variety. For this team to function effectively such a vast range of skills should be utilized in several ways. Firstly it is essential that all team members are kept informed on current developments in their specialist fields. All professionals should be responsible for updating themselves in their own specialty. Secondly, the range of skills and expertise should combine to offer a better standard of care for any individual; and thirdly, by working together it should be easier for these standards of care to be maintained.

These three points will be examined to illustrate how they can be utilized. There must undoubtedly be a shared vision and agreed objective so that the individuals of the team are working towards the same goal. In order to achieve this some members may need to have more input than others. For example, for a housebound patient to continue living at home there would be more input from the district nurse than the practice nurse. Responsibilities should be made clear so there is no confusion over who is meant to be doing what. This will save time and ensure that the team works as an efficient unit. For this to be possible there is the necessary component of communication.

Effective communication is essential if objectives, roles and tasks are to be agreed. Normally this takes place as a result of team meetings. If meetings are not possible for every member, another form of communication must be designed for absent members to receive information to prevent communication breakdown. Whether this involves regular phone conversations or smaller submeetings does not matter provided there is a mechanism in existence that keeps each team member aware of what the others are doing. Communication will be discussed in more detail later in the chapter.

It has already been established that for any team to be effective there has to be commitment to the agreed objective. When this objective is achieved it is important that members are complimented by each other to maintain their interest. Respect for the parts played by individual members in achieving goals should be encouraged. This again returns to the concept that some team members have to provide more input for an outcome to be achieved.

There is no doubt that some form of management is required for effective team function. Within the primary health care team in particular, this management function is complicated (Tettersell *et al.*, 1992). The variety of members required to make up the team suggest that though people may work together they may have different perceptions and ideologies. Knowledge of the individuals in the team is necessary to establish their strengths and weaknesses. As well as the individuality of team members there is also a complex organization management structure.

The GPs effectively manage themselves with regard to employment status. Practice nurses are employed by the GPs but are sometimes managed by one senior practice nurse or the general practitioner, or indeed no one. District nurses and health visitors are health authority employees and thus tend to be managed by their neighbourhood nurse manager. Other members such as community psychiatric nurses (CPNs), dietitians and chiropodists are also responsible to their respective health authority whereas social workers tend to be employed by social services.

This diverse management structure provides the potential risk of the team breaking down. Different managers' views may cause a conflict of ideas. A district nurse manager may have a different view from that of the GP. To whom does the district nurse respond? To the GP who is responsible for the patient or the district manager who is responsible for the nursing care provided for that patient? There is the difference in commitment to the practice rather than just the patient. The CPN will have many patients not on the GP's list. With which patients do priorities lie? The increase in fundholding practices may ease some of these difficult structural problems.

By discussing the concept of team management the subject of hierarchy within the team is highlighted. Some sociologists would argue that hierarchy is a dangerous thing in a team and should be avoided at all costs. However, it can be clearly shown there must be some organizational management within the team for it to function effectively.

Hierarchy within an organization can be described as being either flat or tall. In a flat organizational structure there are few levels of hierarchy whereas in a tall organization there are many levels that separate the lowest positions from the highest. Examples of both are shown in Figure 3.4.

An example of an organization with a flat hierarchy would be a general practice. Flat hierarchies imply a broader span of control in the sense that there are fewer management levels to go through for approval of actions. This, however, also means there are fewer promotion opportunities for its employees. A classic example of this is the practice nurse, although a sense of promotion can be achieved if moving from a small practice to a large one to manage a team of nurses. This tends to be the only scope for promotion.

An example of an organization with a tall hierarchy would be a hospital. Here there are many levels with different specialties reporting to different managers. For example, staff nurses will not report to the same manager as a radiographer but their managers in turn may or may not report to the same manager. This is known as the span of control. Comparing

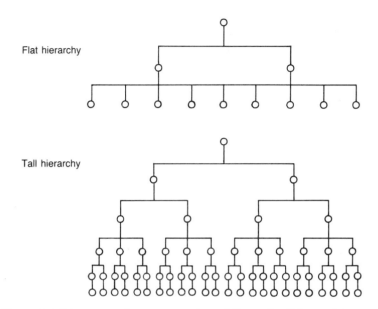

Figure 3.4 Diagrammatic representation of flat and tall hierarchies.

the two organizations shows us how flat hierarchies do have broader spans of control in that most employees are likely to report to just one supervisor; in a tall organization structure, fewer employees report directly to a higher manager and hence the span of control of each manager is classed as narrow. That is not to say that their influence is less.

The concepts of span of control and hierarchy are similar. The fewer the levels of hierarchy, the broader the span of control. It is often noted that communication between levels is improved if there are fewer levels for any message to be passed through. This makes sense in that the time it would take for a message to be passed from the lowest member of the hierarchy to the top member in both organizations would vary greatly. It would obviously be quicker in the flat.

Tall hierarchies are sometimes accused of being less efficient in that decisions are made at the top which may affect members at the bottom without any direct consultation or involvement. This can also happen in flat hierarchies depending on who is the leader. Rules and regulations are built into systems to facilitate control. Normally the larger the organization the more bureaucratic the structure becomes.

LEADERSHIP AND THE TEAM

Is a leader different from a manager? For example, there are leaders who have no management skills but probably most good managers are also good leaders. Some examples of different theories relating to leadership are:

Trait theories

These suggest that leaders are born and not made. Stogdill (1974) identified traits that were consistently associated with leadership; intelligence, dominance, self-confidence, high energy level, task relevant knowledge were among those listed. Trait theories are no longer taken so seriously by management theorists but some organizations still carry out character and personality assessments when looking for their leaders.

Style theories

These are based on the concern for people and the concern for production. They promote the democratic leader (Blake and Moulton, 1964), the idea being that the more democratic the leader the more productive they can be. This notion is associated with the increased involvement required by other team members; the greater involvement causes greater commitment and energy from the group. This democratic style approach is now thought to be too simplistic and other factors should be considered.

Contingency theories

Contingency theories (Lewin, 1951) probably come closest to common experience. Four variables are considered important. The personality and style of the leader; the needs and attitudes of the workforce; the actual requirements of the task; and the organization within which everything is happening.

Michael Maccoby (cited by the Open University, 1988b), a writer in this field, identified four types of leaders. No type is superior to the others and all have their good and bad points. He divided them into four types and likened them to:

The craftsman

The most traditional character, aims to build high quality products. Self-contained and exacting, can become uncooperative and inflexible. He does not build teams, he leads by ordering subordinates to apply what he thinks is the best technical solution.

The jungle fighter

Likes power. Life and work are a survival game in which winners destroy losers. He is calm and protective to his family but ruthless to enemies.

The company man

Orientated to service and institution building, concerned with the human side of a company. Committed to controlling corporate integrity. His identity is based on being part of a powerful and protective organization. He can sustain cooperation from subordinates but he is not daring and lacks the adventure needed to lead innovative organizations.

The gamesman

Takes calculated risks and is fascinated by techniques and new methods. He thrives on competition and is able to hype others up to his excitement level. He may be rash and live in an unrealistic world in which he is prepared to lie and manipulate in order to achieve.

All the above traits can be seen in leaders of any establishment or organization. There are other factors, too, that affect the way a leader works.

Everyone has their own collection of values and experiences and their own ideas on how a leader should act. This will undoubtedly affect the way anyone in a position commanding authority acts.

Another factor is the way people vary in the amount of work they delegate. No one in responsibility delegates to someone who they do not think is capable of performing the task. However, it does take time to build up confidence in work colleagues which is why delegation sometimes takes longer than it should.

Finally stress is an important issue. People react differently to it, some in a positive way, others negatively, so stress may influence leadership styles.

All these issues can be related to the leadership styles used in general practice. To a certain extent they may be used in the way a nurse deals with patients. If the concepts behind leadership are understood it should create a better style of patient management.

COMMUNICATION IN HEALTH CARE

Communication is essential in teamwork to allow for ideas and feelings to be conveyed to fellow members. An effective team member therefore needs to have good communication skills.

The importance of communication can be observed by working out how many people are actually communicated with in a working day. By including writing, telephone conversations and face-to-face consultations, a large list is compiled. Communication is a two-way process (hence the prefix 'co' in communication). Although communication might be assumed to be the mere expressing of an idea to someone else, communication will fail if the person to whom a message is given is not listening and therefore does not receive the message.

Communication can be considered under two headings. **Partial** communication is when ideas have been conveyed and the receiver of these ideas acknowledges them. **Full** communication is when these roles of sender and receiver constantly change (Open University, 1988a). For example, on hearing an idea the receiver does more than merely acknowledge it, as in partial communication, but actively becomes involved in conversation, perhaps using the initial idea as subject matter to express personal ideas or feeling. Full communication is a conversation whereas partial communication may be the giving of a command. People communicate not only by spoken word but also by writing and gestures.

If communicating through the spoken word there are two choices: either face-to-face or by using a telephone where gestures and expressions are absent. Using the spoken word in preference to the written can have certain advantages. Firstly there is the chance for full communication in the sharing of ideas and the expression of feelings. Most people would argue that the spoken word is a more natural and less formal method of communicating and can be more personal as non-verbal communication such as touching can also be used.

Written communication in general practice can vary from graffiti on walls, notice boards and suggestion boxes to the more obvious methods such as letters and memos. The advantages of written communication include the benefits of having something written down that can be used as a reference. It also allows the sender time to say exactly what they want without interruptions and unexpected responses. Memos serve a useful purpose of being able to be circulated to a large number of people who do not have to stop their work to attend a meeting to listen to the same statement and it can also allow for simple and concise instruction.

Non-verbal communication is used alongside the spoken word often without thought. Tone of voice is important. For example, 'Why haven't you taken your medication?' could come across as a concerned question or an aggressive one depending on the tone of voice used. Periods of silence are another method of non-verbal communication. Where, when and how long the periods of silence go on for in a consultation may indicate something important. In face-to-face communication tone of voice and the use of silence are just two ways of communicating non-verbally. Another important factor is body language. People are generally unaware of their body language. What they are saying and what their body is doing may contradict each other.

Communication can often be unsuccessful but knowing about the barriers that lead to bad communication can help to overcome them (Open University, 1988a). Sometimes it is difficult to get the message across. This may be because of uncertainty as to how the target receiver will react to the message: also our own uncertainty may make articulation of the message confused. Alternatively a person may be unclear what they want to say. In verbal communication the message is sometimes changed as the conversation proceeds. This cannot be so for written communication. If a clear message is to be given then time may need to be spent defining it.

Sometimes the written word may be an easier and safer option than the spoken word. If there is a choice in the mode of transport of the message then time should be spent deciding which is the best method. Problems can arise if, for example, something important was not put in writing and there was a difference in opinion after the conversation as to what was agreed.

Sometimes it appears that a patient seems to have deliberately ignored medical advice. However, has he ignored it or did he merely not understand the message? Sometimes it is assumed that the patient is familiar with medical jargon and nurses forget that they are using it because it is part of their communication techniques. There are many medical stories where the patient has followed exactly what the doctor has said but in fact totally misunderstood the meaning. For example, most practice nurses will have been handed a specimen bottle with tap water in it. The doctor's instructions probably were to 'bring a specimen of your water to the surgery for testing' and the patient has done just that.

Sometimes people are unable to communicate because their individual views are poles apart and they will never meet. There is little that can be done in these situations but if any sort of agreement is to be reached, both sides usually have to compromise; people have to agree to disagree.

There are other factors which also affect communication, such as the surrounding environment. If there are lots of telephone interruptions it is very difficult to have an intimate conversation with a patient. Distraction should be kept to a minimum. Another problem in effective communication is that the receiver or patient may sometimes give the answers they think they should be giving and not what their true feelings are. The nurse is sometimes better placed than a doctor in this situation because patients do not seem to feel they have to put on the same act for nurses.

Finally an extract from *The Guardian* newspaper, 22nd February 1983 (cited in Open University, 1988a) highlights how written communication may be misinterpreted and shows the need for care to be taken with all methods of communication.

COMMA COST NURSE'S JOB   A comma cost a nurse, Mrs Angela Penfold, her job, an industrial tribunal ruled yesterday. Mrs Penfold, aged 50, wrote to her health authority in Torbay, Devon, to complain about her senior nurse at a health centre in Bovey Tracey. She said in her letter: 'I have come to the opinion Mrs Pepperell is out to make my life hell, so I give in my notice'. Because of the unintended comma, the health authority took the letter to be her resignation. When the authority later refused to allow Mrs Penfold to withdraw the letter, it was effectively sacking her, the tribunal ruled. Mrs Penfold, who agreed that the letter was worded badly, said: 'I cannot write letters, and I did not word it right. I never intended to resign. I meant that she was trying to get me to hand in my notice'. After deciding that Mrs Penfold, of Fore Street, Torquay, did not mean to resign, the tribunal adjourned a hearing of unfair dismissal.

CONSULTATION TECHNIQUES

The art of good communication is of paramount importance when discussing consultation techniques. By being aware of the barriers to effective communication the practice nurse should be able to avoid certain situations where communication is known to be more difficult. The importance of speaking the 'same language' as the receiver has already been discussed as has the fact that interruptions should be kept to a minimum. There are other techniques that would help improve consultation. Body language can be classed as non-verbal communication. It is used constantly by people without them being aware of what they are conveying. For example, when a nurse informs a patient she has plenty of time to discuss a problem and then proceeds to check the time every few minutes this verbal message is contradicted by the non-verbal cues and clues that are transmitted through body movement.

Alternatively non-verbal communication can serve to reinforce the spoken word (Open University, 1988a). 'Please take a seat' can be reinforced by actually pointing to the seat. This serves to complement the verbal message. Similarly, appropriate head nods and eye movements can signal to another person to continue speaking. However, this can appear insincere if done too often and at inappropriate times.

It is important to mention the environment in which the communication is to take place. For example, the position of the patient's and nurse's chairs in the treatment room may affect how easy it is to communicate. People tend to communicate better if there is no barrier, such as a desk, between them so the positioning of the chairs at a corner of the desk is often more effective. There is an optimum distance for communication known as personal space (Sommer, 1969). Intimate conversations reserved for close personal friends can take place between 0–45 cm apart (Open University, 1988a) but these are unlikely to happen in the treatment room. The next range up is for conversations involving interpersonal information. Again it is usually the space range used by close friends for a personal conversation, generally 45 cm to 120 cm. Anything over 120 cm to 360 cm is the distance range used for interviews and business interactions which would be the expected range for a patient/nurse conversation. The nurse should be aware that some treatment room procedures actually encroach on a patient's personal space and the patient may have difficulty coping with this.

Communication is an essential element to efficient working practice. It involves the people at work and the patients. Nurses should be aware of how to become effective in this field to help them achieve a better working environment.

MOTIVATION

People do the strangest things. There's the athlete who trains by running 120 miles a week. The businesswoman rich enough to ensure she never has to work again striving for more power and money. The Voluntary Service Overseas (VSO) worker giving up the comforts of western life to help those in the third world. Those giving up their time for the good of others and those that would destroy all their friendships for the sake of their jobs. Why? Why do people do these things and how does it impact on the management of a general practice?

As discussed earlier, one of the many qualities of general practice is that it brings together individuals with a range of skills from different social and academic backgrounds. This diversity of personalities, if harnessed correctly, can add real value to the organization but it is crucial to appreciate and identify the differences that exist. In their book *Managing Human Resources*, Eimicke and Klimley (1988) highlight the diversity of personalities and the impact that they have on the motivation of staff. 'Why does one employee toil industriously while the worker at the next desk seems to have lost steam? What makes one employee pitch in willingly during a rush project while another coasts along doing the minimum amount of work? What makes people enjoy working hard?'

Motivation can be defined as morale or a positive attitude towards work translated into purposeful activity (Eimicke and Klimley, 1988). Morale is an immeasurable quality though its importance in the work environment cannot be over-emphasized. By understanding both the personalities of the organization's staff and the theories of motivation it should be possible to tailor the management framework to cater for these individual needs and hence to maximize the morale and efficiency of the organization.

Research has shown that organizations displaying a genuine concern for the well-being of staff as well as productivity will invariably be more profitable, function more effectively as a team, have lower absenteeism and staff turnover and be more committed to creativity and quality. Motivation is therefore a key management concept and some of the key theories on the topic will be considered.

Theories of motivation

As one would expect, a concept that relies on the behaviour of individuals has an enormous number of highly divergent theories. Some of the early theories, for example, were based on the belief that a satisfied worker will be a productive worker or that by offering incentives individuals will make more effort to reach objectives (McGregor, 1960). This may fit the classic model of motivation whereby the 'carrot' rather than the 'stick' will produce the desired results but it is necessary to establish what factors act as incentives. For example, is it money or something different? Unfortunately these are questions which cannot always be answered; what may be an incentive for one individual may not necessarily be so for another.

Douglas McGregor (1960) developed two theories, theory X and theory Y, based on assumptions made by managers regarding their staff. McGregor felt that there were two very contrary sets of ideas as to 'what makes people tick'. **Theory X** is based on the fundamental assumption that people are essentially lazy. They also lack ambition, are indifferent to the needs of the organization as a whole and, perhaps crucially, are gullible. **Theory Y** on the other hand is based on the more positive assumptions that people are both willing and able to work hard, to take responsibility and therefore to contribute to the goals of the organization. They are, however, reliant on management to provide an environment in which personal goals attract the same level of importance as those of the organization and where both sets of goals are congruent.

Obviously theory X and theory Y are based on contrary sets of assumptions of people's personalities and as a result the best way to manage and motivate those people will also differ. Theory X will support the motivation of individuals using coercion and tight control (the 'stick') whilst theory Y highlights the need for management to be supportive of and collaborate with staff.

Most modern literature and work studies on motivation have concentrated on the idea that people are motivated by other factors than purely the economic. These are felt to hold the key to motivation and whilst there may be value in the propositions of both theory X and theory Y, the latter with its more positive assumptions about people is considered to hold the real key to the subject.

Maslow's work (1954) can be used to illustrate that management must provide an environment for staff to satisfy their individual goals by trying to identify and categorize those goals or needs. Maslow believed that people could group their needs into five categories. He also felt that these categories were arranged in a hierarchy so that only by satisfying a lower level need could one move on and try to satisfy a higher level need. In ascending order, Maslow's hierarchy of needs is:

- Physiological
- Safety
- Love
- Esteem
- Needs for self-actualization.

The concept that behaviour is 'needs driven' was taken further in 1969 by Clayton Alderfer. He tried to reclassify the needs identified by Maslow and to simplify them into only three categories.

- Existence needs
- Relatedness needs
- Growth needs

Existence needs are the primary needs. They relate to the basic instincts of survival and reproduction. Relatedness needs are those derived from social interaction such as respect and trust. Growth needs are those such as learning new skills and gaining more responsibility.

It is obvious that the ability to satisfy the primary level needs in either Maslow's or Alderfer's models cannot be the responsibility of management. These are needs satisfied primarily outside the work environment though they may impact on the work environment if they are not being met. For example, a receptionist who feels insecure because of external pressures will probably not gain enough security from the practice to compensate for this but management's awareness of such problems allows them to motivate better with the use of variables they do control, such as ensuring they praise good work and remain constructive if the need to criticize ever arises.

The motivation theories developed on the basis of behaviour being 'needs driven' were still not felt by some to provide the complete answer. Herzberg (1968) suggested that individuals are driven by goals and summarized his views in an article for the *Harvard Business Review*. The article, entitled 'One more time: How do you motivate employees?', developed the theory that motivation fators must be intrinsic rather than extrinsic to the job itself. Whilst accepting the topic was complex, Herzberg still felt the question was a simple one: 'How do you get someone to do something?'.

Initially management felt that force could be used whether it be in the crude form of physical force or in more subtle forms. Herzberg set about demolishing many of the traditional myths about motivation. One theory which held that motivation could be increased by decreasing an individual's work time was negated by Herzberg who simply made the point that motivated staff work, and are happy to work, long hours. On the topic of monetary reward he demonstrated that pay rises only motivate until the next pay rise is due. Likewise the provision of fringe benefits simply help to complicate the management and remunerative system without providing any real evidence that they motivate staff. Other factors all considered part of a healthy work environment such as employee counselling, sensitivity training, management communications and job participation are all believed to have failed to provide the answer.

Herzberg felt that factors influencing job satisfaction and motivation were quite distinct from the factors that provoke job dissatisfaction. He developed his ideas that intrinsic factors relating to a job, such as recognition of achievement, quality of output, responsibility, growth and advancement, are the ones that motivate. Factors which merely avoid dissatisfaction (called hygiene factors by Herzberg) are extrinsic to the job and do not truly motivate. Supervision, relationships, salary and work conditions are all examples. For instance, with this theory, having well paid people working in modern offices is quite clearly not sufficient or essential in producing well motivated staff.

The motivation–hygiene theory argues that efficiency should not be increased by rationalizing. It is better to enrich the work and so create a more effectively utilized staff.

One word of warning; do not confuse job enrichment with job enlargement. The latter simply results in the addition of meaningless and uninspiring tasks to other meaningless and uninspiring tasks. Enrichment adds value to the job and consists of seven key principles.

- Remove controls but retain accountability. The motivators in this instance are responsibility and recognition.
- Increase individual accountability for the work. The motivators are responsibility and recognition.

- Distribute to individuals complete units of work and so highlight their outputs. Motivators are responsibility, achievement and recognition.
- Grant additional authority to staff. Motivators are responsibility, achievement and recognition.
- Make internal reports available to all staff rather than simply supervisors. Motivation is internal recognition.
- Introduce new and more difficult tasks. Motivators are growth and learning.
- Assign individuals specific tasks, allowing them to become experts. Motivators are responsibility, growth and advancement.

(Herzberg, 1968)

Herzberg concluded by pointing out that job enrichment, like all management theory, is dynamic. It is not sufficient to do it once and forget about it; it should be ongoing. He states that the agreement for job involvement can be summed up quite simply: 'If you have employees on a job use them. If you can't use them on a job, get rid of them either via automation or by selecting someone with lesser ability. If you can't use them and you can't get rid of them you will have a motivation problem.'

Herzberg's theories highlight the fact that managers everywhere face the problem of how to motivate their employees successfully. They agree that financial incentives do not provide the answers and that the people must be made to feel that they are carrying out a job worth doing. Managers need to move away from the old fashioned adversarial approach to management and focus on a more participative approach where the concept of the team takes a higher profile.

Typical modern management thinking suggests that authority and discipline do not in themselves motivate. This has been backed up by research and may also have been your own experience when working in the hospital setting, where the nursing management and their techniques do not reflect current thinking.

In conclusion, therefore, whilst accepting that motivation is a key concept in management science and that understanding how to motivate will provide an efficient and productive practice, there is no definitive right answer. Individuals must be appreciated and treated as individuals and some may still respond to the 'stick' rather than the 'carrot', though management theory would suggest that the carrot is preferable. The theories discussed highlight the more commonly held views but not necessarily the right ones in every instance.

Good managers remain flexible and provide frameworks in which the satisfaction of people's individual goals is directed to ensure that the goals of the organization are also satisfied.

QUALITY ISSUES IN THE PRACTICE

Without management guidance it is more important than ever for nurses working in the relative isolation of a practice to be able to assess the standard of their work and improve on it if necessary.

Quality assurance in practice involves the practice nurse being aware of personal (and colleagues') values (Sale, 1990). These values once identified can be used as the standard which the nurse aims to achieve. Therefore it is clear that when assessing and auditing any aspect of work there must first be a desired standard already defined. Current practice should be at this defined level but this may not always be the case. Setting the standard of care and measuring whether this standard is reached are two separate things.

In 1980 the Royal College of Nursing produced their *Standards of Care* document outlining how important standard setting is. A second document, *Towards Standards* (1981), identified prerequisites for successful standard setting. One of the key factors which came to light was accountability. Nurses must be clear about their accountability and guidelines are laid down by the UKCC in the *Code of Professional Conduct* (1992). The basis of this Code is that a nurse, midwife or health visitor is now accountable for their practice. This is a crucial factor in nursing practice. Nurses working in isolation with no other colleagues to turn to for advice must be certain they feel trained and competent to undertake any tasks asked of them.

When a desired standard is planned, the nurse should ensure that it is achievable, observable, desirable and measurable within the *Code of Professional Conduct*.

Having set the standard of care, the next stage is to observe the current practice. For example, if the desired standard of care was to achieve an 80% target figure for cytology uptake, this stage would involve calculating what the true uptake was. It may be as low as 50% in which case the quality of care will not match the standard set. The next stage, having assessed the quality of care provided, is to compare it with the desired standard. It is likely that action may be needed to change the current situation if the standard is to be achieved. Time should be spent identifying a more effective way to reach the standard. It may well be that the standard set is unachievable and hence this too has to be changed.

By constantly reassessing the quality of work, the practice nurse can help ensure that the standard of care is not reduced. Audit is a useful tool to help introduce change. If, for example, a nurse is working in an environment that is resistant to change, it may be influenced by setting an agreed standard of care. Measurement of the standard will show whether it is reached and the change necessary can be highlighted. However, audit is time consuming.

To summarize, audit and quality assurance in general practice can serve to:

- bring the team together to discuss desired standards;
- set the desired standards of any current practice within that team;
- monitor the quality of care given in that practice;
- compare the actual standard with the desired standard;
- interpret findings;
- bring about changes in care that are required to achieve the desired standard;
- reassess the desired standard – is it achievable? – and change it if necessary.

The whole concept of quality assurance rests on practice nursing staff being aware of the roles and standards expected of them. There is much emphasis now on audit in general practice and this should ensure that quality is maintained as all members of staff learn to examine their practice.

MANAGEMENT AND THE PRACTICE NURSE

To return to the original example of setting up a health promotion clinic, it has been demonstrated how basic management concepts are applied in practice.

Initially the importance of the planning stage was discussed. This has been expanded by drawing on Lewin's classic change theory (1951) which highlights the importance of planning. By using this theory any change necessary to start a new project can be identified. Practice meetings, as discussed in both the communication and teamwork sections, also become a crucial part of the planning stage. Already three other aspects of management have been incorporated into this seemingly simple first stage.

The next stage, the motivation stage, was established as an extension of the planning stage. The motivation section explained how all members of staff will have their individual goals and will have their own motivation needs. Every practice will therefore have a different approach to this stage depending on the individuals concerned. Leadership skills also become evident and it is here that leadership and motivation become linked. Poorly led staff will not be motivated. Both of these areas are concerned with the variety of individual behaviours. These differences have to be addressed if there is to be harmony and teamwork within the working group.

The initiation stage of the project again brings in the need for communication skills. Communication techniques are just as important to the nurse as to the doctor. All staff have to be motivated for this stage to succeed, otherwise the system will break down. Teamwork links in to this point because at this stage it is crucial that the team work together.

Evaluation is the final stage before the process starts again. Once again the management concepts that have been discussed throughout the chapter are all integrated into this section. Quality issues come into this stage, whereby the preset standard made in the planning process can be evaluated to see if it has been achieved.

This chapter has illustrated how management theory is related to general practice and is also relevant to the work of a practice nurse. General practice is a business and it is easy to relate the business side of the practice to any other organization. The health care provided by the practice is slightly different. However, it has been established that a large part of management theory directly concerns the individuals involved within the organization. Organizational management is present in every practice. How effective it is now concerns the practice nurse, as it has become a part of her job.

REFERENCES

Alderfer, C. (1969) A new theory of human needs. *Organizational Behaviour and Human Performance*, **4**, 142–75.

Blake, R.R. and Moulton, J.S. (1964) *The Managerial Grid*, Texas Gulf Publishing Co, Houston.

Eimicke, V. and Klimley, L. (1988) *Managing Human Resources: Documenting the Personnel Function*, Pergamon Press, Oxford.

Handy, C.B. (1988) *Understanding Organisations*, Penguin, Harmondsworth.

Herzberg, F. (1968) One more time: how do you motivate employees? *Harvard Business Review*, **46**, 53–62.

Lewin, K. (1951) *Field Theory in Social Science*, Harper and Row, New York.

Maslow, A. (1954) *Motivation and Personality*, Harper and Row, New York.

McGregor, D. (1960) *The Human Side of Enterprise*, McGraw Hill, New York.

Open University Open Business School (1988a) *Communication: The Effective Manager*, Open University Press, Milton Keynes.

Open University Open Business School (1988b) *Leadership: The Effective Manager*, Open University Press, Milton Keynes.

Open University Open Business School (1988c) *Managing Change: The Effective Manager*, Open University Press, Milton Keynes.

Pritchard, P. (1981) *Manual of Primary Health Care*, 2nd edn, Oxford University Press, Oxford.

Royal College of Nursing (1980) *Standards of Care*, RCN, London.

Royal College of Nursing (1981) *Toward Standards*, RCN, London.

Sale, D. (1990) *Quality Assurance*, Macmillan Education, Basingstoke.

Sommer, R. (1969) *Personal Space: The Behaviour Basics of Design*, Prentice Hall, New Jersey.

Stogdill, R.M. (1974) *Handbook of Leadership: A Survey of Theory and Research*, Free Press, New York.

Tettersell, M., Sawyer, J. and Salisbury, C. (1992) *Handbook of Practice Nursing*, Churchill Livingstone, London.

UKCC (1992) *Code of Professional Conduct for the Nurse, Midwife and Health Visitor*, UKCC, London.

FURTHER READING

Huczynski, A. (1991) *Organizational Behaviour: An Introductory Text*, Prentice-Hall, New Jersey.

Kron, T. and Gray, A. (1987) *The Management of Patient Care*, 6th edn, W B Saunders, Philadelphia.

Schemerhorn, J., Hunt, J. and Osborne, R. (1991) *Managing Organizational Behaviour*, 4th edn, John Wiley, New York.

4

An introduction to epidemiology

Colin Stevenson

DEFINITION

Epidemiology has been defined as:

> The study of the distribution and determinants of health-related states or events in specified populations and the application of this study to the control of health problems.
> *(Last, 1988)*

This wide definition recognizes that the modern study of epidemiology is concerned not just with the causes and occurrence of disease but also factors associated with health and with the functioning of health related services. The modern epidemiologist is as likely to be concerned with the results of health care interventions as with the risk factors for diseases.

EPIDEMIOLOGY AND THE PRACTICE NURSE

Sheppard (1992) lists amongst the tasks of the practice nurse the following.

- Promotion of self-care;
- Performing immunizations;
- Giving vaccinations for foreign travel and advice on health care abroad;
- Care of patients with chronic disease in the community;
- Taking cervical smears;
- Audit and self-assessment.

To undertake these tasks does not require a knowledge of epidemiology, but to understand why they are being done does require that knowledge. This understanding makes the difference between a mechanistic approach and an intelligent thinking approach. An appreciation of the causes of disease and critical understanding of the strength of the evidence is required if opportunities for health promotion and disease prevention are to be taken. The clinical care of chronic disease and its complications, including their prevention, is enhanced by a knowledge of their distribution and determinants. The principles of screening must be familiar if a screening programme is to be applied effectively to a population. Clinical audit requires data collection, analysis and interpretation, while an evaluation of the services provided demands the development of valid outcome measures.

HISTORY

Space permits only a very brief examination of the history of epidemiology. Hippocrates referred to the importance of environmental factors as determinants of disease. John Graunt, a haberdasher, was interested in the spread of plague in London and produced *The Nature and Political Observations Made Upon the Bills of Mortality* in 1662. William Farr became the first medical statistician in the Office of the Registrar General in 1839 and developed a classification of disease that was the prototype for the International Classification of Diseases, Injuries and Causes of Death. He also produced Annual Reports of the Registrar General in which public health problems were discussed based on evidence from routinely available data.

The best known episode in the history of epidemiology relates to the work of John Snow on cholera in 1854. Several lines of evidence were advanced for an association between consumption of water from a particular source and the occurrence of the disease. He showed that cholera deaths in an area of London were related to the companies supplying water. In particular, no cases were reported in subdistricts supplied solely by the Lambeth company while many occurred in subdistricts supplied by the Southwark and Vauxhall company. Furthermore, in subdistricts supplied by both companies deaths were much more common in houses using Southwark rather than Lambeth water. Snow was also able to show that the only major difference between affected and unaffected households was their water supply. He also noted that workers in a brewery with its own water supply were unaffected while members of surrounding households died in great numbers. The death of a widow in Hampstead was related to her habit of drinking water specially collected from the affected area. The difference in the two water supplies was their source, Lambeth water being drawn from the Thames upstream of sewage outlets while Southwark water was drawn down-stream.

It should be noted that the vibrio now known to be the cause of cholera was not isolated by Robert Koch until 1883. Koch had published in 1878 his *Aetiology of Traumatic Infective Diseases* where he expounded his postulates, the evidence required to show a micro-organism to be the cause of a particular disease.

DATA SOURCES

Population data

A population is usually defined as a group of persons resident within a geographical area. This definition may be expanded and generalized for some epidemiological purposes to include other subjects, for example health care organizations such as general practices. Residence is sometimes interpreted as physical presence in a location rather than place of abode, for example the concept of a daytime population that includes those working as well as living in an area. The concept of location may be abandoned and another shared characteristic used to define a population, for example a general practice population may be defined as those persons registered with the practice.

Nationally, population sizes are measured by a census when an attempt is made to enumerate all persons usually resident within the national boundaries on a particular day. Between censuses population estimates are produced using data for the three elements of population change – birth, migration and death. Collecting these data is now a responsibility of the Office of Population Censuses and Surveys (OPCS). In Britain a Bill for the taking of a census of the population was put forward but defeated in 1753. The first national census was undertaken in 1801 and the first census which identified individuals was that of 1841. In recent times a census has been conducted every ten years, the latest being in 1991. The considerable effort and expense of the exercise precludes a more frequent enumeration. An accurate account of the population is the prime purpose and questions for possible inclusion are tested to ensure they do not cause offence or inhibit compliance. In recent censuses there have been problems in finding an acceptable question relating to ethnicity, for example. It is a legal requirement to provide information for the census. Trained enumerators are employed to deliver forms and check completion on collection. However, there are concerns as to the completeness of the enumeration, particularly in inner city areas. The significance of this for health is that resources are allocated for health care based on population sizes and their characteristics.

Information that was collected in the 1991 census included the following.

Households
- Accommodation type and tenure
- Rooms and amenities including central heating
- Availability of cars

Persons
- Sex, date of birth, marital status, relationship in household
- Address now and a year previously, country of birth, ethnic group
- Long term illness, employment, qualifications
- Occupation, industry, place of work, hours worked

Registration of births, marriages and deaths began in 1538 but was underaken by the ecclesiastical authorities and was very incomplete. Civil registration commenced in England and Wales in 1837 and, although it became a legal requirement, was incomplete in the early years. Numbers of births and deaths are now accurately recorded. An additional requirement for those attending births is to notify the local health authority and to supply certain data such as birth weight. This notification is used to initiate child health surveillance and birth weight data is passed to the registrar for onward transmission to OPCS.

Population predictions are produced in addition to estimates of present populations but are less reliable. The particular difficulty is the prediction of fertility.

Mortality data

Mortality data are derived from the registrations of deaths. When a death occurs a medical certificate of cause of death must be provided by a registered medical practitioner except that in some cases the death will be reported to the coroner. This certificate is given to the 'qualified informant' who is usually a relative of the deceased but may be a person present at the death, the householder in whose property the death occurred or even a person finding the body. The death must be registered within five days by the informant taking the certificate to the local registrar. The informant is required to give information concerning the deceased, including occupation. Completed death drafts are processed by OPCS and in particular, the cause of death is coded according to a set of rules that should identify the underlying cause of death. These data are used to provide the routinely available information on mortality.

It is important to understand the process involved in the production of mortality data since this is the key to understanding the accuracy of these data and their limitations.

Morbidity data

Routinely available morbidity data come from a variety of sources. The definition of morbidity presents some problems since for many purposes there is a requirement for 'official' certification by a health professional before a person is categorized as ill. Minor departures from a state of perfect health are so common as to be normal; most suffer from headache, indigestion, mild depression or some similar symptoms every few days but they would not characterize themselves as ill. Morbidity data are available from the community, primary care, secondary care and for specially selected conditions.

General Household Survey

This is a survey conducted by OPCS that collects information on many topics from a small random sample of the population. The content is changed regularly so that more topics can be included over time. Questions have been included on episodes of acute illness, chronic illness and disability, use of medications and use of health care facilities. Health related behaviour such as smoking has also been covered. The principal problems with these data are the relatively small number of topics covered and the fact that the picture is a national one that gives no clue as to local variations.

General practice data

The only routinely available data from general practice concerns consultations for infectious conditions that is supplied by a national network of specially recruited practices. These data provide valuable information that supplements that available from other sources such as microbiology laboratories, for example, about the incidence of influenza.

A national morbidity survey of general practice has been undertaken recently at ten year intervals around the time of the census. These have provided valuable data about consultation rates and referral rates for specific conditions. However, there are some concerns that the practices willing to take part in this exacting exercise are not typical. Additionally they do not reflect local variations between practices and populations served.

More information is now being collected by practices as computerization spreads. Much morbidity information is recorded and some is processed either for use within the practice for purposes such as audit or is provided to market research companies who monitor the use of pharmaceuticals. There is some concern that these data are biased towards conditions of particular interest or those consultations involving prescribing.

Hospital morbidity data

Patients presenting in hospitals represent a small proportion of those seeking health care but usually represent the more severe problems. Of these the majority will only attend as outpatients and for this group no routine morbidity data are available. Inpatients and those treated as day cases are a highly selected group that in some specialties such as dermatology are totally unrepresentative of the generality of people attending hospital. Consequently hospital morbidity data must be used with care. In some circumstances these data can provide an accurate estimate of incidence; for example, operations for true appendicitis as opposed to suspected appendicitis provide a good guide to the incidence of this condition. Other conditions such as renal failure in the elderly may never be diagnosed and routine data will be a poor guide to incidence.

Disease registers

Registers are specialized information systems set up primarily to help in the management of or monitoring of specific conditions. They may be national, such as cancer registration, or local, such as diabetic registers. Registers have the following characteristics.

- Based on individuals not episodes of care;
- Relate to a particular condition or set of conditions;
- Based on a clearly defined population;
- Data collected longitudinally, usually at each service contact.

For maximum effectiveness ascertainment should be as complete as possible and therefore larger registers such as the regional cancer registries will employ considerable resources and use a variety of sources such as clinicians, pathology records and death certifications as inputs to the system. Checks are built in to ensure that double counting does not occur and that all cases are followed up. In this way accurate data are available concerning incidence and survival and over time trends can be detected.

District or practice based registers for chronic diseases such as diabetes are assuming greater importance in their management. They can be used to ensure that each known diabetic is following a personal programme of planned care but they also provide data about the incidence of complications of the disease.

Lifestyle data

Apart from some data from the General Household Survey and other national surveys relating to topics such as patterns of food consumption, there are few measures of health related behaviour in the general population. Health authorities have therefore undertaken such surveys on a district or regional basis to identify sections of the population where health promotion interventions would be most beneficial and to monitor the outcome. Topics covered usually include smoking, diet, alcohol consumption, physical activity and sexual activity together with knowledge of other risk factors.

DISEASE MEASUREMENT AND INDICATORS OF HEALTH

Incidence and prevalence

Simple numbers of persons suffering from a disease are of limited value. For most purposes it is desirable to relate these numbers to a population. A variety of populations may be chosen, for example persons registered with a general practice, living in a specific geographical area or present at a particular location during a specific interval. There are two useful measures of disease in a given population. **Incidence** is a measure of newly diagnosed cases within a specified interval. **Prevalence** is a measure of the total number of cases in a population either at a particular time (point prevalence) or over a specified interval (period prevalence).

Comparing rates

A rate on its own is of limited value. There is frequently the need to compare rates for the population of one area or practice with that of another or to consider changes over time. However, populations tend to vary in major determinants of vital events and disease that are in themselves of little interest. The greatest of these is of course age. One approach is to compare age specific rates but this is inconvenient and difficult if it is required to compare all sectors of the population.

Age standardization provides a summary measure allowing for differences in age structure in populations. There are two methods of standardization – the direct and indirect. The direct method results in an age adjusted rate for each population calculated from a knowledge of the numbers in each age group and age specific rates for both populations. The indirect method produces a ratio of observed events in the population of interest with its age structure and age specific rates for the event in the standard population. The best known example of an indirectly standardized rate is the SMR (standardized mortality ratio) used to compare the mortality experience of a population against a national standard such as the population of England and Wales.

Some measures of health

Fertility

The crude birth rate is the number of births per 1000 population. It is affected by the age and sex structure of the population and therefore a more specific measure is preferred.

The general fertility rate is the number of live births per 1000 women aged 15 to 44. Age specific fertility rates are live births per 1000 women within specific age bands.

The total period fertility rate is the average number of live births per woman that would occur if current age specific fertility rates operated over the 30 years reproductive life span.

Mortality

The crude death rate is sensitive to the age structure of the population. Age specific death rates or age adjusted death rates, as described above, are to be preferred. The age standardized mortality ratio is a useful summary measure of mortality providing a comparison with a standard population.

The perinatal mortality rate is the number of stillbirths plus the number of deaths in the first week of life per 1000 total births. It is a useful measure of fetal loss at or around delivery but improved neonatal care may result in babies who would have died previously during this period surviving a few days longer.

Need for statistics

It is not intended to describe statistical techniques here and the interested reader is recommended to consult a standard text of medical statistics. The practice nurse does not require this detailed knowledge but should appreciate why statistics are used in epidemiological studies.

Fundamental to the need for statistics is the mathematical idea of probability. The simple approach to this is to consider a situation with a finite number of outcomes such as throwing an unbiased die. Each of the six possible outcomes is just as likely to occur and therefore each is assigned the probability of one sixth. This does not mean that if the die is thrown six times each number occurs once but if the die is thrown many times then we would expect each number to occur with approximately equal frequency and furthermore, the more times the die is thrown the more equal these frequencies become.

A consequence of this is that if we select any particular sequence of throws we will obtain an estimate of the probability of obtaining any particular number that is nearer to the true value as the length of the sequence increases. This means that if we take a random sample of a population and measure the occurrence of some event in the sample, then how good an estimate this is of the number of events in the total population will depend on the size of the sample. Statistical techniques provide a measure of how good an estimate the sample provides.

One method of doing this is by calculating a confidence interval around the figure for the population estimate derived from the sample. For example, a 95% confidence interval represents the range of values within which the estimate is expected to lie 95 times out of 100. It is often of interest to decide if the occurrence of events in two populations is really different based on observations on samples from each population. We can conclude that results from two samples are really different at a chosen level of probability if their confidence intervals have no common element. The following hypothetical example shows the effect of sample size.

Suppose the incidence of a disease in population A is estimated as 10/10 000 and in population B as 20/10 000. Are these incidence rates really different? The certainty with which the question may be answered will depend on the number of cases observed as demonstrated by the calculation of approximate 95% confidence intervals (see Table 4.1).

Table 4.1 Effect of number of observations on confidence intervals

Number of events	95% Confidence interval
10	5.3–18.8
20	12.8–31.3
100	8.2–12.2
200	17.4–23.0
1000	9.4–10.7
2000	19.6–20.4

Thus it may be seen that while no definite conclusion is possible based on a small number of observations, the difference is much more certain as numbers of observations increase.

EPIDEMIOLOGICAL STUDIES

The practice nurse requires some knowledge of epidemiological studies not because of a requirement to conduct such studies but to understand their significance in the practice of primary care. Only a brief discussion of methodologies is provided and the interested reader should consult a standard text for more detail.

Descriptive studies

Descriptive studies are important because they often form the basis for further studies by providing a hypothesis to be tested. Essentially they provide a description of the pattern of disease. Disease patterns are related to the variables of person, place and time. For example, many diseases are more common in one sex and at different ages or a pattern of disease may be observed in persons who operate a particular industrial process. The observation of temporal and spatial clusters of disease has been important in finding causes; for example, legionnaire's disease.

Case series

Reports of cases have been important in establishing associations between diseases and risk factors. Examples include hepatic angiosarcoma and occupational exposure to vinyl chloride, venous thromboembolism and use of oral contraceptives, and repetitive strain injuries related to occupational and leisure activities. However, one feature of these observations is that the diseases are rare or novel. It is interesting to speculate if the association between thalidomide and congenital malformations would have been recognized if the malformations had been more diverse and more common than phocomelia.

Correlation studies

Correlation studies relate disease and risk factors at the population level. It is possible to show positive relationships between, for example, cigarette consumption and ischaemic heart disease and bronchial carcinoma. However, such studies do not relate individual exposures to disease occurrence. It is also possible to show spurious associations, for example, between ownership of consumer goods and ischaemic heart disease.

Cross-sectional studies

The community prevalence of a disease is often difficult to estimate from routine data and a special survey must then be undertaken to measure risk factors simultaneously. For example, a survey of the prevalence of angina pectoris may include determination of smoking and dietary behaviour. The problem with this type of study is the impossibility of determining the precise sequence of events; that is, if the disease followed exposure to the risk factor. One exception to this is where the risk factor is known not to change over time, for example eye colour.

Case control studies

Case control studies are simple in essence but complicated in practice. The study links known cases of the disease to persons who are thought not to have the disease and then attempts to measure exposures to possible risk factors in both groups. Linkage is by the process of matching and this is commonly done for factors such as age and sex that are not of interest. It must be remembered that it is not possible to draw any conclusions about risk factors for which cases and controls have been matched.

The major problems with case control studies are finding suitable controls and measuring exposure to risk factors. For example, it is often convenient to use hospital patients as controls but they are ill or disabled and their disease may share risk factors with that under study. It is difficult to get an unbiased sampling frame for the general population and securing co-operation may also be problematic. In case control studies the exposure to risk factors is being determined retrospectively and sometimes the cases may be seriously ill or have died. Relatives may have to be relied on to provide an exposure history. It is also difficult to attempt to quantify some exposures; for example, many people cannot give an accurate history of their diet over the past week, let alone several years. Another problem is recall bias where some exposures are more memorable than others or there is a difference in the recall between cases and controls. For example, women with breast lumps will often recall relatively trivial trauma to the breast while normal controls will not.

The advantages of case control studies include the relative ease of their performance, the ability to examine several possible risk factors at one time and the ability to study rare diseases. For these reasons a case control study will normally be conducted first to test a hypothesis.

Cohort studies

It has been customary to use the term retrospective study synonymously with case control study and prospective study with cohort study. However, while it is true that the vast majority of case control studies are retrospective, cohort studies can be either. The retrospective reconstruction of cohorts is a valuable method in occupational epidemiology where there are accurate records of exposures to risk factors.

Cohort studies compare groups who are either exposed or not exposed to a risk factor. Both groups are free of the disease of interest at the start of the study. In prospective studies the groups are followed over time and the incidence of disease is noted.

Cohort studies provide a direct estimate of the risk of disease following exposure but they do require considerable resources to follow the subjects over a period of time. It is important that subjects are not lost to follow-up and the method is only really applicable to common diseases since a sufficient sized cohort is required to produce a significant number of cases.

An example of epidemiological methods

An excellent example of the application of epidemiological methods to progressively confirm and refine a hypothesis is provided by the work on the causal relationship between tobacco smoking and carcinoma of the lung undertaken by Sir Richard Doll and Sir Austin Bradford Hill (Doll and Bradford Hill, 1950, 1952, 1954, 1956, 1964; Doll and Peto, 1976).

In 1950 a preliminary report was published of a case control study that had been set up to examine the relationship between smoking and lung cancer. Previous work in several countries had suggested that the increase in the incidence of carcinoma of the lung might be related to an increase in smoking. Other possible causes such as atmospheric pollution had also been proposed. This preliminary report provided some evidence of the positive association between lung cancer and smoking but was not conclusive.

The results of the completed study published in 1952 showed that men with carcinoma of the lung were more likely to be smokers than the controls and the proportion of heavy smokers was higher in the disease group.

A preliminary report appeared in 1954 of the famous cohort study of British doctors. In 1951 this study had been initiated when 40 000 respondents to a questionnaire had been put into two groups of smokers and non-smokers. This early report based on death in males over 35 showed a positive association between smoking and both carcinoma of the lung and coronary heart disease. A further report in 1956 confirmed these findings and showed a definite dose response effect. It also showed that stopping smoking reduces the risk. Associations were also found between smoking and cancers of the upper respiratory and digestive tracts and with chronic bronchitis, pulmonary tuberculosis and peptic ulcer.

This cohort continued to be followed up and a further report was published in 1964 confirming the results previously noted. A definite positive linear association was shown between amount smoked and death rates for carcinoma of the lung. It also showed that while death rates had increased in the general male population they had declined in doctors. This was attributed to concurrent reductions in smoking in the latter group. It is also noted that air pollution is unlikely to be an important cause of lung cancer.

The further report of the cohort study appeared in 1976 and was based on over 10 000 male deaths. The important features of this study were the completeness of follow-up and the accuracy of the determination of cause of death. It showed conclusively the relationship between smoking and carcinoma of the lung, including a dose effect, and the specific reduction in lung cancer deaths as smoking decreased in the study group. It also showed the contribution of smoking to deaths from other causes such as coronary heart disease, chronic bronchitis and other vascular diseases.

Measures of risk

It is not necessary to understand how risk is measured in epidemiological studies especially as this can be complex for case control studies. However, it is useful to be familiar with the terms used.

Relative risk is the ratio of the incidence of disease in the exposed group to the incidence of disease in the non-exposed group. This can be calculated directly in cohort studies. In cerain circumstances a reasonable estimate of the relative risk may be obtained from a case control study by calculating the odds ratio. This is the ratio of odds in favour of disease in the exposed group compared with the unexposed (Table 4.2).

A relative risk greater than one indicates a positive association between the factor and disease while a value less than

Table 4.2 Ratio of odds in favour of disease in exposed and unexposed groups

	Exposed	Unexposed
Disease	a	c
No disease	b	d

Odds ratio = {a/b}/{c/d} = ad/bc

one suggests a protective association. It is possible to calculate confidence intervals for relative risks and if they contain one then there is no evidence of a relationship either way.

Attributable risk is a measure of the disease in an exposed population associated with that exposure. If it can be assumed that other risk factors are acting equally in both groups the attributable risk may be calculated from the difference in incidence between exposed and unexposed groups.

Causality

Finding an association between a possible risk factor and a disease is not sufficient evidence that the factor causes the disease. Several other relationships are possible. The factor (A) may be associated consistently with another factor (B) which is the true cause of the disease (C). Alternatively both the disease and the proposed risk factor may actually be caused by a third factor.

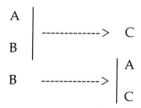

The situation is likely to be much more complicated since it is believed that most diseases are caused by multiple factors that may have complex interactions. An example is the vast number of proposed risk factors for coronary artery disease. Even in apparently simple cases there are difficulties. For example, infection by the tubercle bacillus is a necessary condition for the development of clinical tuberculosis but it is not a sufficient condition since clinical disease does not always follow infection. Clinical disease requires other factors that seem to act on the immune mechanisms.

There are several features that should be considered when deciding if a possible risk factor has a causal relationship to a disease.

- Strength of association. This is often considered in terms of relative risk – the higher the relative risk, the more likely the factor is causal.
- Biological credibility. A plausible biological mechanism is known.
- Time sequence of association. The exposure should clearly precede the disease.
- Dose response. There should be a consistent relationship between dose of exposure and disease incidence but this may not be linear and a threshold value may be evident. Indeed, in some circumstances a low dose may be protective and dose rate may be important. These features are illustrated by the relationship between exposure to sunlight and malignant melanoma.
- Consistency. All studies should provide similar evidence leading to similar conclusions.

Intervention studies

Intervention studies seek to decide if preventive or therapeutic measures influence a disease process. Essentially they compare outcomes between a group given the intervention and a group not given the intervention. However, in practice most studies are much more sophisticated. The best known example is the clinical trial used to evaluate drugs. A detailed description of the design and analysis of such studies is not appropriate but a few features should be noted.

- The study population should represent the general population to whom the results are to be applied.
- All of those chosen to participate in the trial who will be drawn from the study population must be eligible for entry into either arm of the study.

- Allocation to either treatment or control group should be a random process.
- Outcome should be assessed without knowledge of the group to which the subject belongs, i.e. the study should be blind and should be as independent as possible.
- Subjects should also be unaware as to which group they have been allocated, i.e. the study should be double blind. This is especially important where outcomes involve subjective judgements such as pain relief.
- Some studies test a new active treatment against an established one while others test against a placebo.
- It is often possible to include cross-over in the study design, i.e. both groups have the experimental and control treatment but in different orders. This allows within-group comparisons.

It may be considered unethical to randomize patients to active or inactive treatment regimes. However, since by definition the active treatment is of unproven effectiveness it can equally be considered unethical to subject patients to treatment that may confer no benefit but cause discomfort however slight.

PRINCIPLES OF SCREENING

Criteria for screening programmes

Screening attempts to sort those who have a disease, of which they are unaware, from those who do not. Screening tests are not diagnostic and are mechanisms to select individuals for further examination.

Wilson and Jungner (1968) have suggested criteria that should be met before a screening programme is initiated.

- The condition is an important health problem.
- There is a phase in the natural history of the disease before it is symptomatic when it is recognizable by testing (see Figure 4.1).

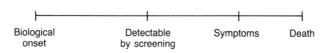

Figure 4.1 Phases in the natural history of disease.

- The natural history of the disease is understood, in particular the phase between the possibility of detection by screening and overt symptoms.
- A suitable screening test is acceptable to the population to be screened.
- An effective acceptable treatment is available.
- Facilities for diagnosis and treatment are available.
- There is an agreed policy on appropriate cases to treat.
- Cost of case finding, i.e. screening, diagnosis and treatment, should be reasonable in relation to total health expenditure and should be continuous, i.e. applied to a population over time, not a one-off procedure.
- Cost finding.

Screening tests

The ideal screening test should identify correctly as positive all of those with the disease and none of those who are healthy. This is theoretically possible, for example, in the case of the prenatal diagnosis of a genetic disorder. However, many illnesses cannot be defined by a dichotomous partitioning of the population. In conditions such as hypertension, illness is

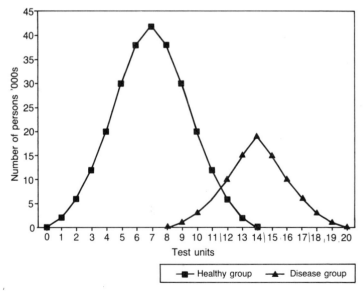

Figure 4.2 Sensitivity of screening tests.

defined by an arbitrary cut-off point in a continuous distribution. It may be supposed that in this situation there are two populations with overlapping distributions (see Figure 4.2).

The performance of a screening test may be measured by determining the **sensitivity** and **specificity** (Table 4.3) **Sensitivity** is the ratio of true positives detected by the test to all those tested with the disease. **Specificity** is the ratio of true negatives to all those without the disease. Ideally these parameters will be both 100%, i.e. there will be no false positives or negatives. However, reference to Figure 4.2 will show this is not possible. If the cut-off point for a normal result is set at eight units then the sensitivity will be 100% but there will be many false negatives. On the other hand if the cut-off is set at 14 units then the specificity will be 100% but many true positives will be missed. In practice the test is likely to operate between these two extremes.

Table 4.3 Sensitivity and specificity in screening tests

	Disease present	*Disease absent*
Test positive	a	b
Test negative	c	d

Sensitivity = $a/\{a + c\} \times 100$
Specificity = $d/\{b + d\} \times 100$

A further parameter is the positive predictive value; that is, the ratio of the true positives to all those found to be positive by the test. Thus, from Table 4.3 we have positive predictive value = $a/\{a + b\} \times 100$. This quantity depends on the prevalence of the disease; the higher the prevalence in the test population, the higher the positive predictive value. Suppose we have a test with sensitivity and specificity of 90%. If the prevalence is 10% then the positive predictive value will be 50%. However, a prevalence of 20% will give a positive predictive value of 69%.

The yield of a screening programme is the quantity of unrecognized disease treated because of the programme. The following factors will result in a high yield.

- High sensitivity.
- High prevalence of unrecognized disease, resulting from high incidence, long latency, long screening interval;
- High population compliance.

PRINCIPLES OF SURVEILLANCE

Epidemiological method underlies the performance of continued surveillance of changes in the health of the population. An analysis of the processes involved was undertaken as a part of a programme to facilitate the development of information systems (Thomas *et al.*, 1992). Surveillance of health status measures the values of selected characteristics of defined populations over time by the systematic collection and interpretation of data. These values are then compared with chosen standards to identify significant differences. Standards chosen may be the value of the same characteristic in another population, e.g. England and Wales, or its value in the same population for a different time period.

Health status surveillance is thus a basis for identifying problems that require new interventions or modification of existing ones to change the values of those characteristics to more acceptable levels – target characteristics.

Surveillance may be established for a variety of health problems, for example coronary heart disease and some of its determinants such as smoking, diet and exercise habits. People known to be vulnerable in terms of health status or recognized as 'priority groups' are commonly chosen as subjects for surveillance, e.g. children under one year, pregnant women, people aged 75 years and over. Populations selected for surveillance should be defined using precise criteria that relate them to location, e.g. children aged under one year living in (district)/(ward)/(region), women resident in (district) attending (hospital) for antenatal care during (period).

Information is produced about the health related characteristics exhibited by these populations. This includes health related behaviour, e.g. attendance for antenatal care, as well as morbidity and mortality. Examples include the stillbirth rate and standardized mortality ratios. On occasions characteristics may be estimated for the population of interest by applying a rate derived from another population; for example, the number of smokers may be estimated by applying rates derived from the General Household Survey. Frequently a population characteristic will be produced from a sample by applying the characteristic of the sample to the whole population from which it was derived. Forecasting a population characteristic, for example by extrapolating trends, is important in deciding future targets.

Population characteristics produced in this way and used for routine surveillance are often available from external sources such as the Public Health Common Data Set or in OPCS publications that provide data at FHSA level.

Examples of topics, relevant populations and population characteristics derived by manipulating data as above that may be used for surveillance are shown in Table 4.4.

Table 4.4 Examples of topics, relevant populations and population characteristics that may be used for surveillance.

Public health topic	Population of interest	Population characteristic
Perinatal death	Children under one week	Stillbirth rate, early neonatal death rate
Coronary heart disease (CHD)	Persons under 65 years	SMR for CHD <65, smoking prevalence
Immunization	Children aged two years	Percentage completed pertussis course Percentage with rubella antibodies
Accidents	Persons >75 years	Age standardized hospital admission rates for fractured neck of femur

Community orientated primary care

Community orientated primary care (COPC) is now beginning to be introduced into the United Kingdom. It has been defined as 'an integration of community medicine with the primary health care of individuals in the community' (Last, 1988). In this form of practice the community practitioner or community health team has responsibility for health care both at a community and at an individual level. Physicians and other health workers who provide primary health care for individuals also endeavour to treat the community as a patient (Abramson, 1983). As described by Kark (1983), its main proponent, COPC is based on an epidemiological appraisal of the health needs of the community and its subgroups and is characterized by the establishment of programmes within the framework of primary care to meet those needs. COPC is practised in Israel, where it has been taught since the 1960s, and in America. Nutting, Wood and Connor (1985) summarize the US experience of COPC in a variety of primary care settings.

The COPC model consists of three components: a primary care practice or programme, a defined population and a systematic process that identifies and addresses priority health problems of the population. The COPC process by which the major health problems of the community are addressed consists of four steps or functions: defining and characterizing the target or denominator population, identifying priority health problems, modifying the health care programme and monitoring the effect of programme modifications (Nutting, Nagle and Dudley, 1991). Nutting (1986) describes each of these functions in terms of five stages of development with regard to the supporting data. The highest stage represents the ideal, where high quality data is available for the activities required to carry out the functions. The intermediate stages describe the activities in terms of different types of data.

EVALUATION OF INTERVENTIONS

Evaluation of an intervention must take place at least twice. Initially it must be shown to be safe and effective during the development stage before it is brought into general use. The principles of intervention trials for this purpose have been outlined above. However, the application of this intervention to a population different to the trial population requires further investigation to ensure that the promised benefits are being achieved in practice. This means that the outcomes of interventions should be monitored regularly. Outcome must not be confused with effectiveness; a good outcome is the result of an appropriate application of an effective intervention.

Outcomes can be measured at both the individual level and the population level.

Individual outcomes are easier to measure; for example, the improvement in mobility and reduction in pain as a result of total hip replacement. At the population level it is theoretically possible to imply a population benefit as a sum of individual benefits but this is difficult to apply to population interventions such as health promotion campaigns. Frequently there is the additional problem of lag time; the desired outcome of the intervention will not become apparent until some considerable time has elapsed following the application of the intervention. This requires the development of valid intermediate measures that are predictive of the final outcome. An additional theoretical problem is that of attribution; is the outcome a predictable direct result of the intervention?

A related problem is that of valuing interventions to provide a rational method of prioritization of those interventions potentially available to the population. The work of health economists has been seminal in this area (Williams, 1974). Measures such as QALYs (quality adjusted life years) have been developed. These are used to measure the outcome of, for example, coronary artery bypass grafting in terms of the extra years gained by the recipient adjusted for the quality of those years in terms of suffering and ability to perform activities (Williams, 1985). However, this approach is not without its critics on methodological and ethical grounds (Carr-Hill and Morris, 1991; Harris, 1987; Smith, 1987). Additionally those measures that have been developed are only available for a few interventions.

CONDUCTING A SURVEY

Increasingly the practice nurse will be involved in or asked to undertake a survey of the practice population. It is not proposed to provide a complete guide here, which can be found in standard texts, but this section will outline the main stages and state some basic principles. These apply to any study, be it one of patient satisfaction with the service or a survey of the health of the practice population.

Main stages of planning

1. Define objective – what is the hypothesis being tested?
2. Read the literature – has it been done before, when, where, by whom and how? What mistakes were made? How can they be avoided? Does it need to be repeated or can the published results be applied? If it has not been done before, something similar certainly has – learn from it.
3. Draft a protocol – define objective, study population and setting and methodology, i.e. data collection, processing and interpretation. Are any permissions required, is ethical committee clearance necessary, should expert statistical advice be sought and is special funding required? Early consideration should be given to the processing and analysis of the data. This must include factors such as the size of any differences it is hoped to detect between subgroups of the study population since this will affect the size of the study population and subgroups.

Data considerations

Data collection requires the development of a suitable instrument, questionnaire or record sheet. The first step is to find out if a suitable validated instrument exists because if it does it is better to use it than invent something new (permission may be required). Examples include the Nottingham Health Profile (Hunt *et al.*, 1986) and the census questions. An additional benefit is that this allows easy comparison between the results from your study population and others to which the instrument has been applied.

If a new questionnaire is being developed, an initial consideration must be how it is to be administered, the basic choice being between a self-completed questionnaire or an interview. The choice will depend on many factors including cost, study population, setting and type of questions being used. For example, a study of an elderly population including open-ended questions would require face-to-face interviews for success. While face-to-face interviews have the advantage of being able to use other information from respondents such as body language, interpretation of replies by the interviewer may introduce bias. Telephone interviews may be seen as a cheaper alternative to face-to-face interviews but are only suitable in certain circumstances and will obviously restrict and therefore bias the study population.

The steps and considerations in the construction of a questionnaire include the following.

- What are the variables?
- What are suitable questions?
- Sequence of questions – start with easy routine questions and leave the difficult and potentially embarrassing ones until later. Use natural links to get a logical progression.
- Questions should be simple, unambiguous and not offensive.
- Make provision for coding.
- Self-completed questionnaires should be attractive and simple to complete with a guide through the questions.
- Include a covering letter signed by the most suitable person and a reply envelope if applicable.
- Consider the need for anonymity or confidentiality.
- Arrange for a pilot trial of the questionnaire on a population similar to the study population.

CONCLUSION

This chapter has provided a basic knowledge of the science of epidemiology and indicated some of its important applications to health care. The following chapters will develop some of these themes and build on this foundation.

REFERENCES

Abramson, J.H. (1983) Training for community oriented primary care. *Israel Journal of Medical Science*, **19**, 764–7.

Carr-Hill, R.A. and Morris, J. (1991) Current practice in obtaining the 'Q' in QALYs: a cautionary note. *British Medical Journal*, **303**, 699–701.

Doll, R. and Bradford Hill, A. (1950) Smoking and carcinoma of the lung. *British Medical Journal*, **ii**, 739–48.

Doll, R. and Bradford Hill, A. (1952) A study of the aetiology of carcinoma of the lung. *British Medical Journal*, **ii**, 1271–86.

Doll, R. and Bradford Hill, A. (1954) The mortality of doctors in relation to their smoking habits: a preliminary report. *British Medical Journal*, **i**, 1451–5.

Doll, R. and Bradford Hill, A. (1956) Lung cancer and other causes of death in relation to smoking: a second report on the mortality of British doctors. *British Medical Journal*, ii, 1071–81.

Doll, R. and Bradford Hill, A. (1964) Mortality in relation to smoking: ten years' observations of British doctors. *British Medical Journal*, i, 1399–1410.

Doll, R. and Peto, R. (1976) Mortality in relation to smoking: 20 years' observations on male British doctors. *British Medical Journal*, ii, 1525–36.

Harris, J. (1987) QALYfying the value of life. *Journal of Medical Ethics*, 13, 117–23.

Hunt, S.M., McEwen, J. and McKenna, S.P. (1986) *Measuring Health Status*, Croom Helm, London.

Kark, S.L. (1983) *The Practice of Community Oriented Primary Health Care*, Appleton-Century-Crofts, New York.

Last, J.M. (ed.) (1988) *A Dictionary of Epidemiology*, 2nd edn, Oxford University Press, Oxford.

Nutting, P.A. (1986) Community-orientated primary care: an integrated model for practice, research and education. *American Journal of Preventive Medicine*, 2(3), 140–7.

Nutting, P.A., Nagle, J. and Dudley, T. (1991) Epidemiology and practice management: an example of community oriented primary care. *Family Medicine*, 23, 218–26.

Nutting, P.A., Wood, M. and Connor, E.M. (1985) Community oriented primary care in the United States: a status report. *Journal of the American Medical Association*, 253, 1763–6.

Sheppard, J. (1992) Partners in practice: the clinical task. *British Medical Journal*, 305, 288–90.

Smith, A. (1987) Qualms about QALYs. *Lancet*, i, 1134–6.

Thomas, J., Holton, S., Jones, T., Parsons, T.T. and Stevenson, C.H. (1992) *Public Health Information Specification: Project Report*, NHSME(E) Information Management Centre, Birmingham.

Wilson, J.M.G. and Jungner, F. (1968) *Principles and Practice of Screening for Disease: Public Health Papers No. 34*, WHO, Geneva.

Williams, A. (1974) The cost-benefit approach. *British Medical Bulletin*, 30, 252–6.

Williams, A. (1985) Economics of coronary artery bypass grafting. *British Medical Journal*, 291, 326–9.

5

Acquiring knowledge of the practice population

Ann Hoskins and Kevin Snee

The aim of this chapter is to help the practice nurse examine the health needs of the practice population using routine information sources.

The chapter is divided into two sections. The first looks at the main sources of routine information. Each source is examined briefly, highlighting the advantages and disadvantages of the information for the practice nurse and the practice population. New developments in data collection in the health service are mentioned briefly. The second section uses four case studies to illustrate the uses of information in health service planning at a local level.

SOURCES OF ROUTINE INFORMATION

Throughout this section the information source is described and some indication of the data's reliability and validity is given. These two terms are commonly used when describing data and it is important to understand them. **Reliability**, sometimes called repeatability, is the extent to which a test or observation gives the same result when done twice under the same conditions. **Validity** refers to the extent that a test actually measures the characteristic that the investigator wishes to measure.

HEALTH STATUS

Mortality information

When a death occurs a medical certificate of cause of death must be provided by a medical practitioner (except in some cases when the death is reported to the coroner). This death certificate has information on the cause of death and other data about the deceased, including occupation. The accuracy of the information depends on the person filling in the form. It has been suggested that there are minor errors in 20% and major errors in 5% of death certificates. The completed death certificates are processed by the Office of Population Censuses and Surveys (OPCS) and this office routinely produces reports on mortality statistics. The information on deaths is linked to other data sources, e.g. population data from the census. This enables comparison between different areas of the country, different age groups and different causes of death.

At this stage it is helpful to give some definitions of the most common death statistics that are used when comparing one population to another, e.g. comparing health districts or wards within a health district.

Crude annual death rate

The total number of deaths during a year divided by the size of the population. This is often multiplied by 1000 so that the rate can be stated as so many deaths per 1000, e.g. 24 per 1000. There are, however, problems with this statistic. An elderly population living in the south of England will have a much higher crude death rate than one of the new towns where there are predominantly young families, which simply tells us that older people are more likely to die. This statistic does, however, give an overall indication of the number of deaths in a particular population and is therefore useful for an initial comparison. There are other statistics that allow us to take account of the different age structures of different populations and therefore to look for other explanations of any differences in mortality. These are given below.

Age specific death rates

Indicate the chances of dying in defined age groups, e.g. number of men dying aged 55–64 years during 1990 divided by the mid-year 1990 male population aged 55–64 years.

There are also cause and age specific death rates. In this instance the numbers of deaths for a specific age group and cause are recorded and divided by the number in the age group, e.g. number of men aged 55–64 years in 1990 dying of coronary heart disease divided by the mid-year 1990 male population aged 55–64 years.

There are special mortality rates for children. Three of the most commonly used examples are given below.

The perinatal mortality rate is the number of stillbirths and deaths within seven days of birth per 1000 total births (live births and stillbirths).

The post-neonatal mortality rate is the number of deaths of live born children after the age of 28 days and up to the end of the first year of life per 1000 live births.

The infant mortality rate is the number of deaths of live born children under the age of one year per 1000 live born babies.

Summary statistics which take account of age and sex structure are as follows.

Standardized mortality ratio

A measure of the number of deaths that have occurred in an area in relation to the number that would have been expected if the death rate for the nation as a whole had occurred in that population. The standard mortality ratio (SMR) takes account of the age and sex structure in a population and its value for the nation is usually set at 100. Thus if an area has an SMR of 125 (all causes, all ages) there are 25% more deaths within it than would have been expected. SMRs also allow comparison of different variables within and between different populations, e.g. sex, age group, social class, particular causes of death. The SMR is an example of indirect standardization. For some indicators direct standardization is used (e.g. health of the nation), but a discussion of the difference and relative merits is beyond the scope of this text.

Potential years of life lost

An alternative way of presenting data on mortality in a population is to highlight the loss to society from premature death, e.g. if a boy aged 15 is killed in a road accident one can say that such a death involves the loss of a considerable number of 'expected years of life'. The potential years of life lost due to a particular cause is the sum of all the years that each person would have lived had they experienced normal life expectation. The normal life expectation frequently used in these calculations is 75 years.

Advantages for the practice population
The information is complete and relatively accurate. Comparisons can be made between different areas, e.g. health districts, electoral wards, and different age groups, e.g. the causes of death in children under one year are different from the causes of death in children one to four years old. These differences can help you understand what you might expect in your population, e.g. if you examine the statistics for an area of similar age structure and socioeconomic situation as your own practice, you can get an indication of the type of health problems that will be prominent in your practice.

Disadvantages for the practice population
Small area data, e.g. for a practice population, are not readily available. Information on electoral wards is available but must be interpreted with caution due to small numbers.

Let us use an example in an imaginary population to illustrate this problem. In this population the number of live births is 2000 and of these 20 die in the first year of life; the infant mortality rate (IMR) is therefore ten per 1000. The IMR will fluctuate such that 95% of the time it lies between 8.7 and 11.3. If, however, we examine a similar but smaller population, e.g. a population with 500 births where five infants die in the first year, the IMR will also be 10 per 1000 but in this instance the IMR will fluctuate such that 95% of the time it will lie between 7.4 and 12.6. Note how with smaller populations the fluctuation increases. One way around this problem of small numbers is to aggregate the statistics for a small population over a number of years (say five or ten); this will reduce the fluctuation but it has the disadvantage of hiding information relating to the individual years. Another technique that is used is moving averages; that is, the value for the year is the average of the values for that year, plus the preceding and following years (in this case the three year moving average).

Mortality information tells us about the diseases and causes of death, but it does not give any indication of the level of suffering in the community, especially in relation to chronic diseases which often do not cause death, e.g. arthritis.

Morbidity information

Morbidity data is available from several sources. The definition of morbidity is difficult as it depends on who defines the person as 'ill' and what is the definition of the illness. There is general agreement about major illness such as diagnosed cancer of the stomach. However, for minor illnesses or complaints which many of us suffer from occasionally there is a problem. For example, when does a person suffering from the common complaint of heartburn start to consider themselves ill and when does their doctor start to consider them ill? There will be marked differences between individuals and even professionals about when to label the person ill.

As with death statistics, it is not enough just to measure the number of people suffering from a disease. One has also to look at the number suffering from a disease in relation to the population under consideration or at risk of getting that disease, e.g. children under five years or elderly adults over 75 years. The terms used to measure morbidity are **incidence** and **prevalence**. These are defined below.

Disease **incidence** measures the rate of occurrence of new cases of a disease in a defined population during a stated period of time, e.g. 56 cases per 1000 population per year. Incidence rates are most useful for acute, short duration illnesses, such as influenza.

Disease **prevalence** measures the number of current cases of a particular disease present in a defined population during a defined period of time. There are two kinds; point prevalence and period prevalence. Point prevalence refers to a point in time, e.g. 170 cases of a disease per 1000 population on the 23rd July 1992. Period prevalence examines the number of cases ever present during a period of time, e.g. 500 cases per 1000 population during July to September 1992. It should be noted that in period prevalence a person could be counted more than once if they have more than one distinct episode of the disease during the specified time. Prevalence indicates the amount of existing disease and is most useful for chronic conditions such as arthritis.

Morbidity statistics are available from the general population, primary care and secondary care. Some of these are based on national programmes and others are based locally.

General Household Survey

This is an annual survey that is performed by OPCS from a small random sample of the population. The questionnaire varies slightly each year so different topics can be examined. There have been questions on the following topics; acute sickness, chronic sickness and use of health care facilities such as consultations with a GP and outpatient appointments.

General practice data

Data on infectious diseases is routinely collected by a national network of specially recruited practices. This data is used to help monitor infectious diseases such as influenza in the community. The National Morbidity Survey of general practice is a survey, every ten years, of morbidity in general practice. Forty-eight practices were involved in the last survey. The practices recorded the morbidity seen in general practice over a period of one year. The morbidity information was linked with other data such as occupation, social class, marital status and area of residence.

Advantages for the practice population
The information gives a picture of the problems nationally, with variation over time. The variation between the particular areas chosen for the study can be seen. The data gives an indication of the morbidity seen in general practice as opposed to the problems seen in hospital and so is more meaningful for the practice.

The practice can compare their statistics on the incidence or prevalence of certain diseases with that of the National Morbidity Survey. This may give an indication of whether the practice is reaching all people in their population who are suffering from a certain disease (the problems of small numbers, however, will also need to be taken into account).

Disadvantages for the practice population
The results of the study cannot easily be generalized to your population, unless the study was carried out in your area.

Different doctors will have different criteria for defining the same disease, which makes comparisons between doctors and between practices difficult because you are not sure you are comparing like with like.

Secondary care data

Hospital data examines the illnesses that get treated in hospital. Only a small proportion of the population with severe illness is treated in hospital. In many hospitals the inpatient data available examines episodes of care for different diagnoses and is not linked to a patient, i.e. ten episodes of care could relate to one person treated ten times, ten people treated once or any combination between these extremes. For some illnesses, however, the data can give an indication of the extent of a problem. For example acute appendicitis only happens once and almost all cases are admitted to hospital. Lengths of stay, staff and expenditures are also collected but these measures are of less use epidemiologically.

Since the introduction of GP fundholding practices it is now possible in many hospitals to link referrals and interventions to specific practices. This whole area of data collection in hospitals is changing rapidly and in future years it will be possible to follow patient flow between primary and secondary care. If the information collected is more patient specific it will hopefully allow better planning that is more sensitive to patient needs. In such systems confidentiality for the patients is of utmost importance.

Outpatient information gives an indication of the numbers attending the clinics but at present, in many hospitals, routine data is not available for specific diagnosis or for treatment given. The information available on outpatients is also developing rapidly and in some hospitals it is possible to have outpatient data that specifies the specialty, the examining doctor and the procedure by the referring practice.

Advantages for the practice population
The statistics are relevant to the local district population and may be compared with national figures. Increasingly the data is becoming practice specific, which will enable practices to compare, for example, their referral rates with other practices which may be useful for audit purposes.

Disadvantages for the practice population
The data is based on what morbidity gets treated in hospital and does not reflect the morbidity in the community.

It has been well documented that hospital statistics are an indication of service availability/demand and not always need, e.g. if no service is available there will be no statistics generated. This does not, however, mean that there is not a need for the service.

The aggregate statistics examine consultant episodes of care, length of stay, etc. It is not always clear what was the exact intervention and indeed the whole area of outcomes of treatment has yet to be tackled.

Disease registers

A disease register identifies individuals with a particular characteristic in common (e.g. a disease such as cancer, mental illness). It is based on a geographically defined area (e.g. cancer registries are set up on a regional basis; some districts have special registers for people suffering from severe mental illness). The information is updated over time, usually at each service contact. There are two types of register.

- Action registers – which are used to identify individuals or families needing an intervention, e.g. cervical smears, immunization, supervision of maintenance therapy;
- Information registers – which are used for collecting information and can be used for research, e.g. cancer registry.

Registers at practice level have many applications, for example in the management of asthma and diabetes and in the management of immunization.

Advantages for the practice population
The registers can be based on local information and can be used to plan local services. Information registers within the practice can help you plan your activities on a daily, weekly and monthly basis. The practice can use the registers to define what level of service or targets they want to achieve. The registers can be used to monitor and evaluate the activities in the practice.

Disadvantages for the practice population
It is very time consuming and often costly to keep a register accurate and up-to-date. If a register is not kept up-to-date those in need may not be targetted or receive the required intervention.

A register often is composed of those people who are in contact with the services. It will not be able to identify those people who have the problem, but are not in contact with services, or those who have not as yet been diagnosed as having the problem.

Other sources of information

Increasingly more and more practices are computerized and there is a considerable amount of information that could be used for planning. Unfortunately not all the information is accurate or reliable and at this stage the data should be used with caution. This is another area of data collection that is developing rapidly and there are at present several pilot projects looking at the feasibility of obtaining reliable accurate data from general practice.

Every general practice has to submit an annual report to their family health service authority (FHSA) giving information about the practice, e.g. staffing levels, activity, etc. and the new regulations for health promotion clinics will also give data that will, in the future, be useful.

Lifestyle and health risk factors

It is important for health promotion purposes to understand the lifestyle and health risk factors of your practice population. Routine data on this is not readily available, though the

General Household Survey does ask questions on alcohol and cigarette consumption.

There are national surveillance systems which give information that is useful for planning. Two examples are:

1. Home accident surveillance system, run by the safety research section of the Consumer Safety Unit of the Department of Trade and Industry. This system collects information on accidents in the home and there is an emphasis on isolating accidents that are amenable to action. The information is collected from a rolling sample of 20 major accident and emergency departments throughout England and Wales. Annual reports are produced and there are several specific reports (such as BMX bikes and electric blankets) and reports on other topics (such as accidents to babies under one year old). The system has also been used for other activities, e.g. legislation, discussions with suppliers, medical research and teaching.
2. Surveillance for accidents at work, performed by the Health and Safety Executive. Annual reports on health and safety statistics are produced.

There may also be local statistics available on accidents at work from your local authority's environmental health department.

Your local health authority may have performed a survey to explore the levels of certain risk factors in the district, e.g. smoking, alcohol consumption, illegal and inappropriate drug use. It may also be possible to compare the data with that collected by your practice, particularly if you are in a practice which is in one of the higher bands with respect to the health promotion contract. (A word of warning: the data will be most useful if you are sure every patient entering the surgery has been asked the appropriate questions and that the data is updated regularly!)

Advantages for the practice population
The national data is accurate and may be relevant to your district. There may be some local surveys that will give an indication of the extent of the problem in your area. These local surveys may indicate the need for multidisciplinary activities or the need for several practices to combine together for health promotion activities, e.g. stop smoking clinics.

Disadvantages for the practice population

The information is usually based on national statistics which do not allow for local variation. Local practice data may not be up-to-date or accurate and is based on the patients that visit the surgery.

It is difficult to get accurate lifestyle information, especially if patients are questioned by a health professional. They know that smoking and drinking are considered unhealthy by health professionals, so when asked by the nurse how many cigarettes they smoke or alcoholic drinks they consume, they often underestimate or deny their levels of consumption.

SOCIAL DATA

Social data can be collected from several sources nationally and locally.

Census data

The census is performed every ten years. On the night of the census all persons alive in the United Kingdom are required by law to be enumerated in the household or other establishment where they spent that night. For this purpose the country is divided into about 115 000 enumeration districts, each consisting of approximately 200 households. (Enumeration districts do not cross ward boundaries, so the statistics from the appropriate enumeration districts can be amalgamated to give statistics for a ward.) For each member of the household information is recorded, e.g. name, age, date of birth, marital status, usual address, relationship to the head of the household, employment status, educational status, ethnic origin, presence of longstanding disability, etc. Every effort is made to ensure the data collected in the census is complete; however there are some concerns about the accuracy of the data, especially in inner city areas.

Population projections for the ten years between the censuses are undertaken by using the census population as a starting point and taking into account births, deaths and migration of the previous year. The data on migration is not accurate and the projections become less accurate with each year after the census.

Certain census variables have been grouped together to give an estimation of the level of deprivation in a community, e.g. the Jarman or underprivileged area score (Jarman, 1983) and the Townsend score (Townsend *et al.*, 1988). These scores have been used to plan services and allocate resources on a basis of need and predicted workload for the GP. The census variables used in these two scores are given below.

- The Jarman score uses eight weighted variables according to how much they are thought to increase the workload of GPs. The variables are old people living alone, children under five, single parent households, unskilled people, overcrowded households, people who have moved house, ethnic minority households.
- The Townsend score uses the four variables unemployed people, households with no car, households not owner-occupied, overcrowded households. These produce a Z score. The average electoral ward in the area scores 0. Any ward with a negative score is less deprived than the average and any score above 0 is more deprived than the average.

Advantages for the practice population

The data is accurate and reliable to enumeration district level, i.e. approximately 200 households. The data can be used to build up a picture of the social structure of the practice population, e.g. housing tenure, unemployment, income levels, births outside marriage.

The data can be used for comparison with other districts. These differences may be important when you are looking at the services necessary for your population, e.g. the services needed by a population where there are many single parent families will be very different from the services needed by a population of pensioners living alone in poor housing conditions.

Disadvantages for the practice population

The population projections become less accurate in the years furthest away from the last census. Inner city practices may have less accurate population statistics.

The practice population will usually be spread over a wide area crossing several wards, thus no ward will completely represent the practice population. This is particularly applicable to city practices.

Registration of births, deaths and marriages

Births, deaths and marriages are registered with the local registrar who is appointed by the local authority. The data collected is collated centrally by OPCS. The recording of births and deaths is considered accurate and the data collected is linked with other data available. For example, birth is linked with birth weight and other social characteristics of the mother.

Local sources of social data

The local authority planning departments, other statutory and voluntary organizations, police, churches and local community groups will all have information that will help you understand the problems in your local community; for example, outbreaks of food poisoning, number of home help visits, free school meals, crime rate, local traffic accidents, etc.

Advantages for the practice population
The information will be locally sensitive and in many cases up-to-date. The information can be directly applied to your population especially if the survey has been performed in your area. The local groups can also give you information about services available from other statutory and voluntary organizations in your area.

Disadvantages for the practice population
The accuracy of the data will depend on how the information has been collected. The information may not always directly relate to the practice population. The information may not always be directly relevant to the health problems that you see in your area, or the solutions to some of the problems are outside the remit of the health service.

HEALTH RESOURCE DATA AND OTHER USEFUL INFORMATION

It is important to understand not only the social characteristics and health problems of your practice population but also to be

Information on health status

Mortality: overall mortality rate, age and sex specific mortality rates, perinatal and infant rates.

Morbidity: incidence and prevalence of specific physical and psychological illnesses: acute (such as food poisoning, measles and meningitis) and chronic (such as ischaemic heart disease, dental caries and depression).

Lifestyle and health risk factors: smoking rates, alcohol consumption, participation in physical exercise, illegal and inappropriate drug use.

Health protection measures: uptake of cervical and breast screening, contraceptive use, use of seat belts.

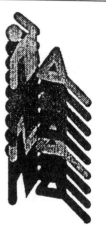

Possible sources of information
1991 census figures
OPCS mortality tapes
Korner data
Regional and district health authority information units
Community health services authorities
Community health council
Previous surveys in the area by a university or a polytechnic

Information sought on availability, accessibility and use of health and social services

Hospitals: location, services available

GPs: location, surgery hours, use of deputising services, number of partners, services offered

Dentists: location, out-of-hours availability

Pharmacists: location, out-of-hours arrangements

Opticians: location

Community health services: chiropody, dental, immunisation, child health, well woman, family planning and dietary services: numbers, locations, hours of operation, and so on

Health visitors, district nurse, school nurses: numbers, services provided

Long term accommodation, sheltered housing, Part III accommodation, nursing homes: number of places, location

Voluntary agencies: services provided

Home help: services available, organisers

Social work support

Receipt of benefits and pensions

Availability of free nursery school places

Possible sources of information
District health authority information units and annual reports
Family health services authorities
Community health council
Local authority departments of social services
Local council of voluntary services
Local office of the Department of Social Security
Local community groups

Information sought on demographic and social characteristics

Age
Sex
Ethnic origin
Marital status
Place of birth
Family and household structure
Income levels
Education: level attained, receipt of higher education grants, receipt of free school meals
Housing: tenure, conditions
Car ownership
Occupation/unemployment
Access to amenities: leisure, shopping, transport
Availability of social support
Personal and domestic security, incidence of crime

Possible sources of information

1991 census plus updates and projections
Local authority planning department
Other statutory and voluntary agencies
Local community groups
Police
Churches
Previous surveys in the area

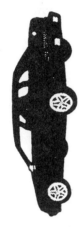

Information sought on the physical environment

Levels of air pollution
Noise pollution
Street pollution
River pollution
Domestic water purity
Local industry

Possible sources of information

Local authority environmental health department: routine monitoring of pollution levels and complaints received from the public
Water authority: routine monitoring of river pollution
Previous surveys

Figure 5.1 Types of information sought and specific sources (reproduced with permission from Sainsbury *et al.*, 1991).

aware of the availability and accessibility of the local services. This will involve compiling data about the local organizations in your area and also mapping out the availability of the services, e.g. accessibility, opening hours. It is also crucial not to forget the resources **within** the community because there may be active community groups in your area. These groups can be very helpful for specific problems you may have in your practice. They also usually have good local networks and can help you contact the appropriate group or person for your problem. Other facts useful to your work include access to local amenities such as leisure facilities, shopping and transport. Information on local industries, levels of noise pollution, street pollution, etc. can give valuable insight into the quality of the local environment.

CASE STUDIES

CASE STUDY ONE   THE IDENTIFICATION OF AN APPROPRIATE POPULATION

The identification of the appropriate population is of fundamental importance because it is impossible to adequately ensure an intervention is effective if it is based on a small unrepresentative sample.

The aim of the project was to review the management of asthma attenders and non-attenders at an anticipatory care clinic. First of all it was important to identify all known asthmatic patients in the practice. Usually, no one database will give a complete picture. If there are several databases available then it may be better to use them all. In this instance three databases were used. The computerized patient register was used to identify any registered patient diagnosed before January 1992. The practice computer system was supplied by AAH Meditel and incorporated the Read clinical classification hierarchy – asthmatics were identified through the disease chapter, filter groups and Read codes (Chisholm, 1990).

A list of patients was then compiled detailing name, address, date of birth and sex. The asthma clinic register was used to identify asthma patients who had attended the clinic between August

1990 and January 1992. This list was then compared manually with the computer generated list. PACT (prescribing analysis and costs) data is available in quarterly returns and comes in three levels from the prescription pricing authority via the FHSA. It is a record of every prescription given out by the practice. Individuals cannot be identified but the number of prescriptions given for asthma therapy was used to estimate the number of asthmatics. With the help of FHSA information, pharmacist, (GP liaison) level 3, reports on the respiratory system prescribing data were obtained for each quarter from August 1990 to February 1992. These data were then used again with the help of the information pharmacist, to crudely estimate the likely number of asthmatics. This was felt to be important because of doubts about the quality of data entry onto the computer database.

The numbers obtained could be summarized as follows:

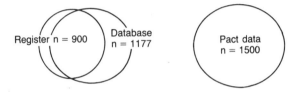

Figure 5.2

There were 60 asthmatics known to the asthma register but not recorded on the practice computer and 277 asthmatics known to the computer but not known to the asthma clinic. Therefore 1237 named asthma patients were identified. The prevalence of asthma for the practice at that point in time was then identified using this figure.

Prevalence of asthma per 1000 practice population
= 1237/12 100 × 1000
= 102 per 1000 population

The estimate from the PACT data was likely to be an overestimate, therefore the true figure for asthma in this practice would lie between 1500 and 1237. Having identified reasonably accurately the total population of asthmatics it is then possible to look at a number of questions such as how effective is the service in offering appropriate and accessible care? How well are patients managed? Are protocols followed? What do patients want out of the service? What percentage of the practice population who are asthmatics does not attend clinics and why? And so on. Some of these questions will be easy to answer using information from the practice database; others will be more difficult and will require an additional study using epidemiological methods such as a case control study (see Chapter 4).

This case study was derived from:

Werne, M.J. (1992) A review of the management of asthma through an anticipatory care clinic: an investigation into the role of an asthma clinic in primary care. Unpublished dissertation for the MPH, Liverpool University.

CASE STUDY TWO   TO DETERMINE THE EFFECTIVENESS
OF A WELL MAN CLINIC

When considering this question you may choose to consider those who attend the clinic and look at them in relation to:

- their compliance with treatment, e.g. do they return to clinic as requested?
- their improvement in health as measured by certain outcomes such as weight loss;
- the amount of pathology diagnosed.

Before doing that it is important to identify whether those who are invited actually attend.

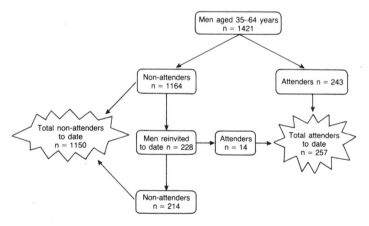

Figure 5.3 Identification of the target group and uptake rate.

The identification of the target group and their uptake rate is of vital importance in the determination of the effectiveness of a service.

We can see that in the example in Figure 5.3, only 18% of the total sample had attended at their first invitation and only 6% of those reinvited had attended. The objective of the investigation that followed was therefore to determine what factors prevent patients from attending a well man clinic and to ascertain whether there are characteristics in the group of non-attenders that differ from those who attend. The sampling frame was all men in the practice aged 35–64 who had been invited at least once to attend the clinic.

The medical records were reviewed to ascertain whether there were any differences between the two groups. Ninety-three were found to have either moved or registered with another practice. A further 32 were deemed unsuitable for a variety of reasons, e.g. they were female, already seeing a doctor, etc. Of the remaining 89 men, 57 were interviewed. Most were aware of the well man clinic but time constraints were a major factor in non-attendance. Attenders were found to be more likely to report taking exercise, to have a healthier lifestyle and to be in paid employment than non-attenders.

Simple administrative problems are often a major cause of a poor uptake rate for a service.

This case study was derived from:

Parry, A.M. (1992) Attenders and non-attenders at a well man clinic. Unpublished dissertation for the MPH, Liverpool University.

CASE STUDY THREE USING WARD BASED DATA TO STIMULATE COMMUNITY INVOLVEMENT

Introduction

Ward based data can be useful for stimulating discussion in a local community. This may then act as a focus for community development activity. The project outlined explains an approach to this that was conducted in Liverpool.

The Vauxhall area has a long history of deprivation. Based in Liverpool's docklands, Vauxhall's social structure has its roots in impoverished, predominantly Irish Catholic, migrant workers. Employment in the area has traditionally been unskilled labour of an insecure nature. Many of the large scale manufacturing industries have been forced to streamline operations or close. The ward has experienced a loss of population of over 30% in the last decade and it now has the fourth highest unemployment rate of all Liverpool wards.

At the same time there has been a large amount of positive activity in Vauxhall. Large scale migration has led to the clearance of large areas of old substandard housing and initiatives such as the Eldonian Housing Co-operative, where a group of residents organized and, despite local authority opposition, succeeded in establishing a new housing estate based on the needs and specifications of the local community. There are also many voluntary and community groups operating within Vauxhall, providing education, support and services for different sectors of the community.

Liverpool family health service authority (FHSA) has used the UPA8 or Jarman Score to identify its eight most deprived wards. A deprived area strategy has been developed aimed at improving primary health care services where health is worst in the city. The strategy focuses on the achievement of minimum standards in general practice and weighted resource allocation by the FHSA. A further key component is the aim of developing community based models of needs assessment and 'bottom-up service development' (Liverpool FHSA, 1991). In Liverpool the Jarman score ranges from − 11 to + 62. Vauxhall has one of the worst Jarman deprivation scores in Liverpool with a score of 46. In all eight wards, because of the high Jarman scores, GPs are given additional payments for providing a service for those patients – this is in accordance with national policy.

The overall aim of the project was to establish a health agenda in collaboration with the local community. This work is based on the belief that specific causes of ill health in the community can be recognized and acted upon by the dissemination of information to, and the direct involvement of, the local community. Evidence from other projects in the Mersey region lends support to this assertion. (Snee, 1991; Croxteth Area Working Party, 1983). There were two main objectives: to provide information for the local community, local practitioners and the FHSA on the health and deprivation in Vauxhall; and to initiate debate and action on health within Vauxhall.

What information was used?

The first stage of the project was to gather together all the relevant data on social deprivation and health in the area (see Figure 5.4).

Social data: household population (size, distribution, change over time), type of housing, unemployment, free school meal status, number of illegitimate births, Jarman data, number of home help visits, crime rate, Townsend scores, higher education awards.

Health service data: standardized mortality ratios (all deaths, malignant neoplasms of lung, myocardial infarction, hypertension and vascular disease, respiratory disease), fertility rate, % low birth weight, perinatal/postnatal rate, stillbirth rate, abortion data.

Health resource data: number of health promotion clinics in area, spells in hospital per annum, inpatient ratio, vaccination/immunization rate.

Environmental data: level and type of local industry in the area, type of complaints to the Environmental Health Department.

Directory of community resources: leisure, shopping, transport, community groups.

Figure 5.4 Data on social deprivation and health in the area (Townsend *et al.*, 1988).

A report was compiled for Vauxhall residents and for professionals involved in the area, highlighting areas of need. The main part of the data was collated from the small area database produced by Mersey regional health authority, although other sources of information were also used, including Merseyside Transport Ltd and Liverpool City Council. The information in the report included both Townsend and Jarman measures and the information in Figure 5.4. Information about community resources in the area was also included.

It is important to recognize and identify community resources that can be used to address the needs identified.

The purpose of this was to include community groups in the data collection and report writing of the project, to form a useful directory for residents and professionals and to establish links for the dissemination of information.

By involving the audience in the processing of the data, e.g. writing the report, it will be more readable and relevant to that audience.

The process, from the initiation of data collection to the publication of the final report, took four months. During this stage dates were established for a series of meetings in the area. Prior to the publication of the report 5000 leaflets were produced for distribution amongst the residents of Vauxhall to give information about the report findings and to advertise the public meetings. It was decided to use existing community networks to disseminate the information so leaflets were given to community groups for distribution and placed at strategic points throughout the ward such as GP surgeries and tobacconists.

The identification of community networks is vital for the dissemination of information and the stimulation of community activity.

The leaflets and the report included pictures drawn by local children about health. A press release was issued which generated publicity through the local newspapers and radio stations.

The second phase of the project started with the public meetings. There were separate public meetings to cover the geographically and politically distinct areas within the ward. All the meetings were held within the same week at well known, accessible local venues. The attendance at the meetings was variable. One area of the ward had developed its own housing co-operative with the support and involvement of a Liverpool based housing co-operative and central government.

The format of the meetings was a welcome and explanation of the work to date, a ten minute presentation of the facts included in the report by one of the researchers and each person was given a copy of the report. It had been intended that the meetings would break up into workshops so that people could all participate more freely. However, people clearly felt safer in numbers, so following the presentation there was a group discussion in which those attending were invited to give their feelings on the health of the area and their views on the particular problems of Vauxhall ward. In all three meetings there was lively debate. The discussion focused on problems in primary health care provision, women's health and environmental problems at the two larger meetings and on particular housing problems at the smaller meeting.

At the end of each meeting informal contracts were given to each of those attending, allowing different levels of commitment to be made, for example an undertaking to distribute information or to become a member of a health forum.

What was the outcome?

One month after the public meetings the first health forum meeting was convened. There were ten people present who were either residents of Vauxhall or professionals directly involved with the local community. At the second meeting 21 people attended. The group was facilitated in the first ten meetings by a facilitator who has experience in community development work. The group are now considering priorities and an agenda for health action in the area. It was important at the end of the first meeting that the forum should consider the plans for the proposed appointment of a vocationally trained GP who will undertake further research with the community in the first year and then become a GP in the Vauxhall area. This is crucially important because it is an FHSA funded project; influence should start there before expanding to develop a more multiagency approach. A job description for this post was written with the group, the job advertised and an appointment made. The local group has been closely involved in the selection and interview of the candidate.

It is important that community activity is channelled at first into issues that are readily achievable and within the remit of the sponsoring organization.

Problems of this approach

GP populations do not fit neatly into a particular geographical area so any policy development which impinges on practice populations may need to be agreed with several practices.

Because there was an emphasis on obtaining a demonstrable outcome relatively quickly there was a lack of community involvement at the earlier stage of data collection. A few key members of the community were kept in touch throughout; however, the most important component of community involvement has now commenced with the launching of the health forum.

The limited involvement of medical professionals was in part by design because it was felt important to allow local people to take the key role in moving the project forward, although some health professionals did attend the first series of meetings and subsequent meetings.

Using existing community networks can have benefits in that it is possible to reach members of the community at a greatly reduced cost. However, they can also operate in an unorganized way and if committees change then co-operation that was previously expected may disappear. It is therefore important to allow extra time to take account of such unforeseen changes.

An alternative structure, i.e. the forum, was established. This was done with the co-operation of key elements of the local community. This was thought to be necessary to bring together the different factions of that community. This does, however, involve bypassing directly elected members of the local authority. Again this was felt to be necessary because certain sections of that community are alienated from the local authority.

This case study was derived from:

Mawle, P. (1991) *Vauxhall Health Report – A Report on the Health of the People of Vauxhall Ward, Liverpool, November 1991*, Liverpool Public Health Observatory, Liverpool University.

CASE STUDY FOUR   RELATING WARD BASED INDICATORS TO PRACTICE POPULATIONS

Much of the data that are collected routinely comes from ward level. It is possible to approximately translate ward based data into practice population data by employing an approach that was used in Cheshire.

As part of the statutory duty of all GPs, annual reports containing a certain degree of information concerning referrals to hospital, staff qualifications, practice formularies, etc. must be made available to their FHSA. In Cheshire the FHSA has compiled the data and made them available to general practitioners in the county so that they can compare their performance with that of their colleagues. At present this has a limited validity because the data supplied are often inaccurate and difficult to relate to other ward based data. Clearly when GPs compare the performance of their practice with their peers locally it is important to take account of the differences in age structure and deprivation in particular. Age structure can be taken account of by using standardization (see Chapter 4), but unemployment or the Jarman score can be taken account of crudely by assuming that wards are homogeneous, i.e. that social indicators are evenly spread throughout the ward. This was done in Cheshire where the following process has been used:

Step 1
Obtain the percentage of each practice's population that comes from wards A, B, C, D.........Z.

Step 2
Multiply this percentage by each Jarman score for each particular ward.

Step 3
Add each resulting number together to give a composite Jarman score.

Worked example

Dr X's practice has 10 000 patients who are drawn from ten wards as shown in Table 5.1.

Table 5.1 Worked example of Dr X's practice

Wards	Population	Percentage of total population (%)
1	3,000	30
2	2,000	20
3	1,000	10
4	1,000	10
5	1,000	10
6	500	5
7	500	5
8	500	5
9	250	2.5
10	250	2.5

Steps 2 and 3

Ward	Percentage of total population (%)	Jarman score	Contribution to overall score
1	30	40	12
2	20	25.6	5.12
3	10	3.7	0.37
4	10	5.9	0.59
5	10	1	0.1
6	5	− 5.8	− 0.29
7	5	9	0.45
8	5	− 6.0	− 0.3
9	2.5	20	0.5
10	2.5	− 10	− 0.25
Total	**100**		**18.29**

Therefore in this instance the composite Jarman score is 18.29.
    This approach can be used for a range of ward based data to make them more practice specific.

Methodological issues

This approach assumes that a group of patients coming from a particular ward has the same demographic make-up as the ward as a whole. There is no easy way to confirm this but it is likely that sometimes this will not be true, particularly where wards are large geographically as is often the case in rural areas. To some extent the problem can be resolved by using enumeraton districts (subsections of the ward for which census data are aggregated); however this is more time consuming and probably not practical at practice level.

Where you know that your population from a particular ward is different, e.g. where there is a nursing home and all of your patients from that ward are from that nursing home, then this method should be used with caution.

ACKNOWLEDGEMENTS

The authors would like to thank Mandy Wearne, Alwyn Parry, Phaedra Mawle, Julie Bradley, Julie Hotchkiss and Susan Ellerby for the use of material upon which the case studies were based and Mark Pickin for proof reading.

REFERENCES

Chisholm, J. (1990) The Read clinical classification. *British Medical Journal*, **300**, 1092.

Croxteth Area Working Part (1983) *Report of the Working Party Appointed to Consider the Needs of the Area.* City Solicitor's Dept, Liverpool City Council.

Jarman, B. (1983) Identification of underprivileged areas. *British Medical Journal*, **286**, 1705–8.

Liverpool Family Health Service Authority (1991) *Deprived Area Strategy.* Liverpool FHSA, Liverpool.

Sainsbury, P., Pursey, A. and Hussey, R. (1991) Neighbourhood watch. Compiling a health profile of an area. *Nursing Times*, **87**(33), 66–8.

Snee, K. (ed.) (1991) *Dallam on Health: A Report of the Steering Group*, Dallam on Health Group, Warrington.

Townsend, P., Phillimore, P. and Beattie, A. (1988) *Health and Deprivation: Inequality and the North–South Divide*, Croom Helm, London.

FURTHER READING

Donaldson, R.J. and Donaldson, L.J. (1993) *Essential Public Health Medicine*, MTP Press, Lancaster.

Morrell, D. (ed.) (1988) *Epidemiology in General Practice*, Oxford Medical Publications, Oxford.

Pickin, C.M. and St Leger, S. (1993) *Assessing Health Need Using the Lifecycle Framework*, Open University Press, Milton Keynes.

Smith, A. and Jacobson, B. (eds) (1988) *The Nation's Health: A Strategy for the 1990s*, King's Fund Publishing Office, London.

6

Needs and the truly reflective nurse

David Seedhouse

INTRODUCTION

As part of the drive to create an independent profession, some nurses have recently shown interest in the idea of 'the reflective nurse'. This chapter considers, through the example of the difficulties of one practice nurse, how the thinking of a 'truly reflective nurse' might develop.

In order to reflect on work situations and problems to greatest effect it is not enough merely to ruminate in an unguided way. It is better to adopt a philosophical approach and so to take guidance from a discipline which throughout history has developed a great variety of techniques and methods for efficient reflection. In what follows, just one of the vast range of philosophical tools is outlined. This method might be called 'reflection on language'. Its purpose is first to see what the users of certain words actually mean and secondly – through deeper reflection – to argue for more precise and considered meaning and so ultimately for better practical work.

THE FRUSTRATED INNOVATOR

It has not been a good day for Christine. As she drives home from the health centre she mulls over yet another rejection and feels deeply weary. It was not such a radical idea. She knows of other practices which employ osteopaths and acupuncturists, so why not this practice? Why would the GPs once again not listen to her proposals? Patients say they would use complementary therapists, many people are helped by such non-medical interventions and the therapists themselves would be glad of the work. Perhaps it is because she is 'only a nurse'. Perhaps the doctors feel threatened. Perhaps they have been so overwhelmed by their schooling that they have lost all intellectual flexibility. Perhaps all they want is a quiet life and conformity guarantees it. Whatever the reason, Christine feels thoroughly dissatisfied. She does not care whether nursing is a 'profession in its own right' or not, but she does need to have a job where her independence and imagination have a place and where her ideas are at least given a chance.

But it is not happening. With each rebuttal of her suggestions for improvement in the health centre's work she has felt more and more ostracised. Over the past year, through various questionnaires and 'discussion papers', she has demonstrated such problems as unnecessary prescribing; arrogance by some doctors during consultations; unintentional discrimination against the least educated patients; too much effort spent on 'running a business' at the expense of 'caring'; and insufficient attention to the 'life problems' of the practice list. In response she has recommended the regular involvement in the health centre of a range of complementary therapists (the proposal which was rejected out of hand this afternoon); guest 'practice lectures' by experts in philosophy, sociology and the history of medicine (open to all staff and patients); peer review of consultations selected at random; patient review of the same; seminars on 'the role of commerce in caring', and public meetings on 'the future of the health service'.

None of these ideas has been found 'appropriate' or 'relevant' by the 'health care team'. It seems that nothing Christine says is taken seriously. Is her position so frail that nothing will work? Is there anything else she can try?

THE POWER OF WORDS

Feeling utterly undermined, Christine calls a friend for advice. Should she leave the practice? Would things be any better elsewhere? Is there anything else she might try at the health centre? Christine's friend used to be a nurse – and so understands the health care world – but has given it up to study humanities at university. She has been pleased to find that she is beginning to think more clearly and has become particularly interested in the use of language. She has a suggestion. It's a long shot but she does not think that Christine has much more to lose at the surgery. Why not focus on the words that are bandied around each day? Why not pin the doctors down and ask what they really mean?

Unlikely as it may seem, careful thinking about words can eventually produce practical improvement. The only way in which human beings convey meaning is through some arrange-ment of signs or symbols. Language is our only route out of ourselves, but – just because it is everywhere – we hugely underestimate its importance. If we wish to change things we tend to prefer direct action rather than to take the time to clarify the meaning of the words we use. But, in the long run, clear thinking can be the more effective strategy.

There are plenty of vaguely used words for Christine to choose from: 'health service quality', 'zero-defect nursing', 'health gain', 'health outcome'. Why not take a piece of health service jargon, take advice and then use decent definitions to argue for change? Since Christine's most common complaint is that 'the needs of patients' are not being met why not examine 'needs assessment'? What does Christine's statement actually mean? Which needs? How many needs? What sort of needs? Who says? By taking the time to examine definitions carefully, by dissecting statements in order to study each component, it is possible to answer such questions systematically.

This is a classic philosophical method but is not unique to philosophy. In fact it is exceedingly common. Versions of it appear in science, in clinical history taking and diagnosis, in solving management problems and even in creating recipes in cooking. The task, in every case, is to turn a muddled picture into something more definite, where the constituent parts can be analysed separately. This is exactly what a scientist does when using a centrifuge machine and exactly what a good cook does when eating a new dish in a restaurant. The inquisitive cook scrutinizes the food, examines the type, amount and combinations of ingredients and having gained a clear picture of the components of the recipe, thinks again in order to try to grasp the cooking process carried out on each ingredient, as well as the order of preparation. This is precisely what a philosopher does with words. Of course, just as a cook takes time to learn necessary skills, philosophical expertise cannot develop overnight. But, like good cooking, it can be learnt and is often best understood through example.

PHILOSOPHICAL HELP

Christine's friend knows of some philosophical analysis on the meaning of 'needs' and promises to put something on paper after she has discussed it with her teachers and colleagues. Three days later Christine receives her friend's advice. Her paper considers 'needs assessment' through an exploration of meaning and so demonstrates one of the methods a 'truly reflective nurse' might adopt. In so doing, it assists Christine with her immediate problem and also helps her begin to foster deeper powers of reflection.

NEEDS ASSESSMENT

Instructed by government to 'assess needs', many managers and doctors have been seeking a definition. But despite several years' labour no sensible account of 'need' has emerged from the health service. The absence of a plausible explanation of need provides an opportunity for truly reflective nurses to create their own definitions and so to encourage progress in directions of their choosing. Naturally it is too much to expect practical health workers to become expert in philosophical analysis overnight but they do not have to think alone. There is much clear, incisive writing available, although few in the NHS know about it.

'What is a need?' has been debated in social and political philosophy for years, in the course of which understanding has grown considerably (Miller, 1976). Drawing on the work of several philosophers past and present a Swedish academic, Per-Erik Liss (1990), has outlined a number of alternative definitions of need. In so doing he demonstrates a tried and tested method of philosophical analysis which, with practice, a nurse might adopt.

Liss' approach to the question 'What is a health need?' is a classic example of one philosophical method. His first move was to survey the literature thoroughly. During this search he picked out key definitions and theories wherever they were clearly stated by an authority. Where they were not he looked for significant themes and patterns and gave identities to them.

Liss found four accounts of need especially significant, naming and explaining them as follows.

- *Ill health* On this account a health need exists if and only if some deficiencies in health exist which require medical care. So if a patient has an infection which requires treatment with antibiotics then it is correct to say that she needs the antibiotic. But if she does not know how to exercise properly she does not have a health need because lack of knowledge is not a health deficiency.
- *Supply (or 'benefit')* This notion insists that effective treatment or care is a necessary condition for the existence of a health care need. Accordingly the way to assess health needs is to undertake a review of present services and then to work out how best to supply these services to 'meet need' most effectively.
- *Normative* According to this view needs do not depend only upon what can be done for a person, but can be brought into being by expert judgement. This means that a need for health care can arise when the assessor believes that health care ought to be provided. For example, if it is decided that screening services should be offered to groups of people then it follows that the specified group of people have a need for health care. Conversely, if it is decided that people over a certain age should not be screened then they do not have a need for health care.
- *Instrumental* In contrast to the other three, this explanation argues that rather than look at what now exists (either as an illness, a service or a point of view) the key to understanding need is to ask 'What state is desired?'. Once the desire has been specified, a goal exists. Then, whatever means are necessary to achieve that goal become the need. Health care, whether it is available or not, is the label which is given to the means necessary for a person to reach the 'health' goal desired.

The NHS currently uses the first three definitions (Stevens, 1991; Johnston and Hunter, 1991; Buchan *et al.*, 1990). Each has apparently been chosen in order to preserve the status quo rather than for its philosophical merit. The intent of all three is to assist practical policy making within the health service, but none could be described as neutral. Each statement is weighted towards existing health service practice. For instance, if 'health care need' is the 'ability to benefit from health care' (currently the most popular NHS definition) then present health care services define what is needed and planners are able to concentrate exclusively on the allocation of available services. With this definition there is no need to compare existing services with potential alternatives. Under the influence of the 'benefit' definition, rather than begin with the neutral question 'What does the population need most of all?', managers can ask 'How might our health care services be used to benefit the population, and so meet their needs?'. The first question requires analysis and policy making from scratch, while the second adapts the meaning of 'need' to match what is currently on offer.

The 'ill health' definition of health care need

The ill health view of health care need has meaning only within a health service system which perpetuates a restricted understanding of 'health'. Only those cases of ill health which the system defines as its concern are said to 'need' health service help. As with the 'supply' definition, 'health care needs' are defined by what the 'health care system' has come to be and what it has come to do. At a stroke the definition limits the extent of the 'health service' to the scope of 'medical services' (which, incidentally, are not defined by the NHS either) and so helps ensure that the health service continues to supply predominantly medical treatments and expertise.

The supply or benefit definition of health care need

On this definition the existence of effective treatment or care is a necessary condition for there to be a 'health care need'.

Thus it follows that the way to assess 'health needs' is first to review services and second to see how they can be targetted most effectively. However, although this definition is 'state of the art' in the NHS, and can be used to justify the redistribution of badly managed resources, it has deep conceptual problems.

Expressed in full the 'supply' or 'benefit' definition of 'health care need' says:

> A person has a health care need if he or she is able to benefit from health care. Conversely, if a person is unable to benefit from health care then he or she does not have a health care need.

Spelt out like this it is difficult to take the proposal seriously. It is one thing to say that a person has no need of useless services but quite another to say that a person cannot need what she cannot have. The idea is bizarre. It would mean:

1. If a person has HIV or AIDS then – in 'commonsense' – he has several health care needs. He may need palliative therapy, he will probably need advice on preventing infection and he could certainly benefit from a cure. But – in NHSese – the AIDS sufferer does not, and by definition cannot, need a cure. He cannot need one because no such thing exists. If a cure were to be available tomorrow, then he would have need of it. But not today.

2. If the existence of 'health care' is a necessary condition for a person to have a 'health care need' then:

   (a) In the past when there were less 'health services' (assuming these to be the equivalent of 'health care') there was less 'health care need'. And in the far past, when there were no useful 'health care services' (if this ever was the case), there were no 'health care needs'.

   (b) In the present, in the least prosperous nations where there are fewer 'health services', there are fewer 'needs for health care'.

3. If 'health care need' is defined only as the ability to benefit from 'health care', as health services expand

and as developments in medical technology and pharmaceuticals continue, so such increased provision 'creates need'. By definition, the more useful health services there are (even if they are only slightly useful), the more 'health care need' there is. Consequently it is theoretically impossible to 'reduce need' by 'meeting it' with more services. Quite the opposite.

The consequences of the supply definition of need are therefore ridiculous. As what can be supplied changes, so need changes but this is 'looking glass' logic, topsy-turvey and back to front. The definition has gained favour not because it truly makes sense, but because it fits with NHS precedent.

Apparently the supply and ill health definitions support themselves nicely. Where the ill health approach runs into problems (for example, it cannot by itself talk of 'the need for health promotion services') the supply definition offers solutions (if 'health promotion' is a beneficial health care service currently provided then it must be a 'health care need'). But this incestuous arrangement is justified only if the NHS is the sole means by which 'health needs' might be met. And of course it is not.

The normative definition of health care need

'Normative' judgements about 'need' are made constantly in the health service. Every time a doctor makes a decision to prescribe or not, he or she is 'assessing need'. Without such judgements it is hard to see how the health service, or indeed any professional service, could function. But just because 'normative judgements' are often required for practice this does not necessarily mean that they are always appropriate or best. Firstly, the 'expert' can be wrong. In fact it is quite normal for 'experts' to differ widely in their judgements about what is needed. Secondly, the 'expert' perception of what is needed can be different from the recipient's view. 'Normative needs assessment' can offer no help in resolving such differences, other than to insist that the patient is mistaken. Thirdly, in common with the other NHS definitions, 'normative' judgements reinforce the status quo. And of the three, the 'normative definition' is the most blatant. It is quite explicit that those who the health service designates as experts are entitled not only to assess needs, but actually to say what 'needs' are. And as the 'experts' do this, so it is virtually certain that more of the services which they judge necessary will be supplied. And if (as is normal) the assessors are expert in medical 'ill health', the nature of what is supplied will reflect that knowledge and those interests. And so it goes on. Each NHS definition offers support to the others (even though, logically, they cannot always be used simultaneously). And each is deeply conservative, protecting what the NHS happens to be at the time.

Analysis of the three NHS definitions of 'health care need' reveals that:

1. 'Needs assessment' is controversial. Alternative definitions of 'health care need' coexist and the 'right' one is not obvious. Choices have to be made and so require justification both within and beyond the health service.
2. Each definition limits the range of 'need' which it says the NHS should address.
3. Each definition is seriously flawed. Yet if 'need' is to be used as a criterion for rationing health care, then rational analysis, from as objective a perspective as possible, is surely morally required. If 'need' is to be used as an NHS tool then, just as with drug dosages and machine specifications, technical accuracy must be a required standard. On the other hand, if 'needs assessment' is an inherently vague procedure then the nature of this vagueness must be clearly demonstrated. If there is more than one way of assessing need, then openness about the reasoning behind 'needs assessment' is imperative.

For those concerned to innovate and to provide new services, the three NHS definitions (as currently used) are virtually worthless. No survey of a health service, or a health centre, carried out under their influence will ever create policy to meet needs for which there is currently no provision, unless 'the experts' are original thinkers.

The instrumental definition of health care need

Because this is not usually the case in the health service, and because there is no philosophically sound way to identify the needs of the users of the service, Liss prefers the instrumental definition. In contrast to the other three options the instrumental alternative is open-ended. It allows the definition of need in accordance with the interests of the patients rather than the traditional purposes of the system. In this way it allows for creative thinking and innovation. For instance, if a survey shows that patients would like alternative therapies or help with budgeting or social support groups, then it can be said that an instrumental need exists. As it stands, without a clear specification of health care purpose and so of the limits of health work, the instrumental definition is open-ended. But this may be seen as an opportunity rather than a problem for the practice nurse who wishes to take more account of her patients' interests.

And it is precisely this situation in which Christine finds herself. In her view the services offered by the health centre do not properly match the needs of the people who use it. But, because she has been told to use a version of the 'benefit' definition of need for her 'needs assessment' work, all her assessments confirm the usefulness of the centre's services and she is unable to conclude that something more is required. Immunizations are done, blood pressures are taken, patients are screened for hypertension, prescriptions are offered and accepted and medication is given for problems caused by bad housing or smoking or 'unwise' sexual activity. These services are taken by the people, therefore – particularly according to the 'supply' definition – the people's needs are being met. But Christine thinks this is reflection in a straitjacket. With the benefit of her friend's philosophical help she understands this more clearly and feels better equipped both to express the difficulty to herself and to articulate it to others. She sees that current 'needs assessment' makes use of a combination of the 'benefit' and 'normative' definitions of need and neglects the 'instrumental' version. But if the aim is to help people with the needs they perceive to be most important, then it is the instrumental definition which ought to be applied.

TURNING THEORY INTO PRACTICAL CHANGE

The test of theories is their application. To judge if the 'instrumental definition' will produce better results Christine decides to review previous cases where she has felt that important needs have not been met. Can she now use her fresh interpretation to persuade the GPs to improve the centre's practice? To find out she leafs through her case diary, thinking again about 'needs assessment' in the cases she recalls.

Flicking through the pages of her diary she finds:

Tuesday

Today we invite people over 60 to come to the surgery for a health check. Each person sees a doctor, the nurse practitioner, the practice nurse, the social worker and a dental therapist. Their physical, mental, emotional and social conditions are assessed by this team and they are given appropriate advice or help.

It is normally assumed by health professionals that the screening of a well population for factors that may eventually produce disease can only be a good thing. By and large I expect they are right, but I wonder whether enough information is always given to the person being screened, on the nature of the risk factor discovered, the chances of its producing some serious illness in the future and the options open for treatment?

Taking patients' blood pressure is *de rigueur* these days, since hypertension is known to cause heart disease and strokes. But the treatment of hypertension is a complicated business. It sometimes involves medication, but it can also include advice to lose weight, exercise programmes and the reduction of dietary fat. Stress control may also be indicated. Do health professonals always ensure they can offer alternatives or adjuncts to medication when screening for hypertension? Since one of the purposes of (practice) nurse care is health education, I feel reasonably happy that I can offer non-medication help with the control of risk factors and I like to believe I am honest with the people who consult me. A recent addition to our screening routine has made me less confident about my commitment to honesty with patients. We have introduced a questionnaire to screen patients for senile dementia. This is thought to be a problem that may be hidden from the GP. Relatives have been known to cope with the effects of a dementing elderly parent until the problem overwhelms them.

I find it difficult to say to people who appear to be mentally perfectly normal! 'I'd like to ask you some questions now to see if you are becoming demented'. Instead I use some euphemism, such as 'Can I ask you some questions to see if you are getting more forgetful?' The questions themselves are embarrassing:

'Where do you live?'
'Who is the present sovereign?'
'When did the Second World War start?'
'Can you count backwards from 20 to 1?'

It's like a school test; is it demeaning to these elderly people?

Sometimes I alter the words or phrases if I think people won't understand – there are many elderly people in this area who left school aged 12. Instead of 'Who is the present sovereign?', I say 'Who is on the throne?' and am not taking the test entirely seriously.

I wonder if the results of the tests are valid. Maybe I'm sending home hundreds of dementing elderly people to leave gas on or wander their neighbourhood after dark?

I ask my colleagues about the test. One says that when she administers it she doesn't say what it is for. The other doesn't worry about it at all. Is it right, I wonder, to tell 'white lies' when to tell the truth might cause problems that could be avoided? Notwithstanding this questionnaire, today I feel I've helped someone.

An 86-year-old man came from screening today. I asked him if there was anything particular I could help him with. He told me he had no relatives and was concerned about ... Here, his voice faltered, so I prompted him, 'about ... ? 'Well', he said, 'You know ... after I die ... ' The man literally had *not one* living relative and was, as he put it, worried about 'the disposal of the dead ' – in other words, his funeral arrangements. I was not sure what he should do, but with the man's consent I contacted local solicitors who gave us advice.

A few days later he came back to see me to collect a booklet I'd ordered for him called 'What to do when someone dies'. He was cheerful and seemed relieved to be sorting out this problem. (From Stilwell, 1989.)

REFLECTION IN ACTION

On studying her thoughts about her work on this Tuesday, Christine sees how her technically unformulated concerns take much clearer shape under a more structured understanding of needs. She focuses on three issues which occurred to her that day: the assumption that screening is a 'good thing', the query over whether enough information is being given and the provision of alternatives to medication (or lack of them). Now she is able to see how different forms of 'needs assessment' have major implications for practice. If she can explain this and have her argument accepted, then future practice at the health centre may change and may come to be based on clear policy rather than precedent and fudge.

Examples

She takes a pen, ponders the three issues in turn and writes down her interpretation of them under the different definitions of 'need'.

The assumption that screening is a good thing

On the ill health account, the intervention carried out on well people (who do not appear to be suffering 'ill health') should not have been done, since on this definition no 'health need' exists. According to the supply view, since the service is available, it must, therefore, be 'needed'. Yet strangely enough, if it were not offered it would, by the same definition, not be needed. Normatively, the 'need' for screening comes into being if experts say such a 'need' exists. And instrumentally there is a need if the patients have the goal 'to be screened'. But this is precisely the issue for Christine. The only way in which the patients can meaningfully say 'I want to be screened' is if they are informed and educated about the screening process. If they are not then they are left in the dark, do not know what they need and so are not in a position to say what they need (and it is this which bothers Christine most). If patients' involvement and understanding are considered important then she sees that she must argue for 'instrumental needs assessment', in clear preference to the other options.

Is enough information given?

On the ill health, supply and normative definitions of 'need', it does not matter how much information is given. It may not even matter if no information is given, so long as the clinical 'need for screening' is met. Only if 'information-giving' is clearly an essential feature of health care, or if the experts agree that information supply is a vital part of health work, can information be said to be needed. Instrumentally the question is 'Do patients desire information – is the possession of the facts a goal for this patient?'. If it is, then there is an instrumental need for information.

Have adequate alternatives to medication been provided?

If medication is being considered then it can be assumed that 'ill health' (in the standard sense) exists. However, the ill health account says nothing about what sort of 'medical care' might be needed, just that some will be if 'deficiencies in health' exist. On examining the supply definition Christine is interested to see how what is *normally given* for a problem inevitably becomes the *natural* and *accepted* thing to do. The logic is this:

We have beta-blockers, these are effective to treat the problem (although there are side effects), therefore the medication must be needed. Since this medication is clearly needed there is no point in considering other therapies.

In other words, what is established as conventional becomes what is thought to be needed. But this sort of thinking can only come out of an ossified system and is exactly the source of Christine's worry. As a truly reflective nurse she decides to argue for the two other definitions of need and the methods of 'needs assessment' associated with them. Armed with the confidence gained through increased philosophical clarity the practice nurse offers her own normative needs assessment and argues that medication should always be the last resort (regardless of what drugs are available) since other methods (such as relaxation therapy and advice on change in lifestyle) are equally or more effective and have fewer clinical side effects.

The following week Christine reinforces her opinion by applying the instrumental definition. She takes a group of patients and offers them a programme of education which candidly explains risks, benefits and the various treatment options. Her aim in making this teaching available is to bring the patients as close as possible to her own level of understanding (which she regards as a normative need of the patient group). This, she believes, will have the effect of enabling them to assess their own needs instrumentally. Christine thinks that by doing this there is a chance that the supply of services will change – and will do so in a manner which involves the users. In this way, through her encouragement of reflection in others, the truly reflective nurse can develop a coherent body of 'needs assessment' theory and technique to bring about desirable change to an otherwise inert system.

Armed with clear thinking and favourable patient responses, Christine attends the next 'team conference'. How convincing will she be now?

CONCLUSIONS

Whatever happens at the practice meeting Christine will have begun to move forward. By considering an example of deeper reflection about the meaning of need and through her own efforts to be as clear as possible about the alternative definitions and their implications, Christine will have discovered a more fundamental form of reflection. If she is to move yet further on, if she is to learn more techniques of reflection, she will need additional philosophical help. The best way forward for Christine would be to study the techniques more formally and so learn more of what the discipline of philosophy has to offer the nurse.

And this applies to nursing in general. If nursing is to demarcate itself as clearly as possible from the medical profession it needs to develop meaningful strategies and expertise which doctors do not have. Through the collective study of philosophy nurses will gain in two major ways. Firstly they will come to understand that reflection is an expertise with clear techniques which can be learnt and secondly they will develop the intellectual power to challenge unclear thinking wherever it is found.

REFERENCES

Buchan, H., Gray, M., Hill, A. and Coulter, A. (1990) Needs assessment made simple. *Health Service Journal*, **100**, 240–1.

Johnston, I. and Hunter, D. (1991) Towards moral rearmament. *Health Service Journal*, **101**, 28.

Liss, P. (1990) *Health Care Need: Meaning and Measurement*, Halso-och Sjukvarden i Samhallet, Universitet i Linkoping.

Miller, D. (1976) *Social Justice* Oxford University Press, Oxford.

Stevens, A. (1991) Needs assessment needs assessment . . . *Health Trends*, **23**, 20–3.

Stilwell, B. (1989) Diary of a nurse practitioner, in *Changing Ideas in Health Care*, (eds D.F. Seedhouse and A. Cribb), John Wiley, Chichester.

FURTHER READING

Seedhouse, D.F. (1994) *Fortress NHS*, John Wiley, Chichester.

The dynamics of practice nursing

Sarah Luft

INTRODUCTION

This chapter seeks to raise awareness with regard to the changing role and the increasing demands that are likely to be expected of the practice nurse. The themes addressed include:

- the development of the discipline of practice nursing;
- the role of the practice nurse;
- the influences emerging from the practice organization;
- the application of a model to practice nursing;
- the thinking practitioner.

At appropriate intervals key points are highlighted which serve to bring together some of the pertinent issues for consideration by the practice nurse.

Hobbs and Stilwell (1989) suggest that the earliest record of a nurse employed by a GP is in Easington, Northumberland, in 1913 and her name was Mary Hannah Robson. Certainly in the early years of this century GPs regularly carried out domiciliary operations and in this work they were assisted by the nurses working on the district. On reflection it is easy to see how the medical advances of that time influenced the shape of nursing generally, so the education needs of nursing primarily pursued a medical focus.

As nursing became accepted as a 'respectable' occupation in its own right, its development was inevitably influenced by the philosophical thinking of the times. Bevis (1982) draws attention to four specific eras – asceticism, romanticism, pragmatism and humanism – and it is suggested that in some ways all of these are present to some degree in nursing today. In the mid nineteenth century when asceticism was the dominant philosophy, nurses were seen as selfless, devoted to duty and hard work and they paid great attention to their patients' spiritual health. In the early years of the twentieth century this thinking gave way more to the romantic era where nurses enjoyed a handmaiden relationship with doctors. Probably this era was reinforced by the occurrence of two world wars, because the third era referred to by Bevis, that of pragmatism, emerges after the inception of the National Health Service and this thinking underlines the importance of the task. Patients were referred to as 'the appendix in bed 11', for instance. The emphasis at this time was on task orientation. From the 1960s there has been more emphasis on the humanistic approach where the nurse views the patient/client as central to any care planning.

Considering the four areas of thinking which influence the goals and values of nursing it can be seen that they are reflected in practice nursing today to a greater or lesser extent. The asceticism philosophy may be the least influential with the other three more prevalent. Modern general practice can foster a nurse/doctor relationship which reflects the romanticism era; task orientation from the pragmatist era can also be seen alongside the efforts to work in partnership with clients and patients which promotes a humanistic perspective.

The National Health Service Act 1946 looked to providing health care for all, which was free at the point of delivery. GPs remained an independent body and the community nursing services were under the control of the local authority – this resulted in a general lack of communication and collaboration between the two. During the 1950s GPs worked single-handedly with some reception help which may have included nursing duties. The Gillie Report (MoH, 1963) identified the lack of communication between GPs and community nurses and a key consequence of this report was the attachment of nursing staff to general practice. Also at this time, the government provided various financial incentives for GPs to form group practices and this concept of teamwork was reinforced by the emergence of health centres.

The pilot schemes which introduced the attachment of community nurses to general practice in general produced favourable reports. Both doctors and nurses enjoyed the increased contact and communication and it is likely that this experience resulted in the 1970s being the decade in which practice nursing really began to emerge, although Reedy *et al.* (1980) suggest that at this time practice nursing was not seen as a 'career' move for nurses.

Probably the next turning point for practice nurses emerged with the publication of the Cumberlege Report (1986). A key proposal here suggested that the financial reimbursements for the employment of practice nurses should be phased out. Her controversial argument focused on problems concerning fragmentation/duplication of care in the community because of the various nurse disciplines involved. She concluded that community nurses could enter into working contracts with GPs and provide the required services. However, neither the GPs nor the practice nurses themselves supported this view. The focus on practice nursing at this time meant more attention was paid to the provision of courses and practice nurses were encouraged to attend the short approved English National Board Statement of Attendance courses which were becoming more widely available.

The next landmark which influenced the development of practice nursing was the implementation of the GP contract (DHSS, 1990) whereby GPs were given specific health promotion targets to achieve and which also related to the generation of income for their practice. GPs could not easily carry out these requirements without further assistance and the number of employed practice nurses increased yet again.

Key points highlighted

- The goals and values of all nurses are influenced by the current thinking of the time. What thinking is in vogue within general practice today? Are practice nurses concerned with the empowerment process whereby they encourage patients to make their own informed decisions? Are they influenced primarily by economic considerations? Do they take on board the concept of the multidisciplinary approach to care?

- The evolution of practice nursing over the century has been surprisingly slow with developments only occurring seriously over the last two decades. However, the last decade in particular has put practice nursing firmly in the area where they are no longer an isolated cluster of nurses, but a professional group capable of working as equals alongside other health professionals to provide a high standard of care within the community setting.
- Doctors and nurses can enjoy healthy working relationships which work for the benefit of the patient/client. The general practice setting is an ideal place in which to nurture this relationship.
- Practice nurses are ready for the educational foundations which will assist them in further professional development.

THE NATURE OF THE PRACTICE NURSE ROLE

It was during the 1960s in the USA, according to De Young (1981), that an acute shortage of physicians occurred, especially in rural and ghetto settings. It was suggested that if nurses had increased skills in assessing the difference between normal and abnormal, could improve their interviewing skills and become acutely aware of health teaching then the care of the child in rural settings would be improved. This idea set the stage for the advent of paediatric nurse practitioners and created the impetus of the 'practitioner' movement as a way of increasing health care to areas where physicians were in short supply.

Bolden and Tackle (1989) point out that in the UK there has been a strong resistance by the medical profession to the development of the nurse practitioner. They suggest that arguments have centred around anxieties expressed where erosion of the GP's role may ensue as a result of this development. Taking this concern a step further we could be looking at the concept proposed by Pearson (1983) who has attempted to promote the role of the nurse as an autonomous practitioner (independent of medicine) in relation to those groups of patients whose primary need is that of nursing rather than of medical care. For nurses working in general practice, this would necessitate categorizing the type of intervention required very carefully.

The nature of general practice is such that it is the medical focus that is currently dominant. Nursing can complement this focus but it could be suggested that for practice nurses, autonomous practice independent of medicine is not feasible at this time. However, there do appear to be avenues opening up in general practice where nurses are able to work on a practitioner basis. An example of this could be in the emergence of an increasing number of nurse run clinics. Once practice nurses have acquired the specialist knowledge and skills required in the management of a specific disease, they may be in a position to offer the practice population an enhanced service. This equates well to the principle under-pinning the practitioner experience in the USA because hopefully the outcome would be not only an improved service, but the provision of that service to a greater number of people.

For nurses to become autonomous practitioners they need to gain confidence in the area of decision making. Research carried out by Mackay (1992) into interprofessional relations between doctors and nurses in hospitals suggests that the doctors felt that nurses lacked decision making power because 'nurses administer the prescribed treatment'. There is every reason to assume that this principle transfers into community settings such as general practice and basically this means acceptance of a power relationship. Mackay refers to the difficulties which ensue in 'obeying orders' especially for those nurses who see their role as prescribing nursing care. On the one hand nurses are subservient to the doctor, but on the other hand they plan a programme of care that they consider appropriate for the patient/client. Perhaps it is worthwhile to consider what is nursing and what is doctoring in general practice and to review these components, utilizing the follow-ing case study scenario.

Mary is 46 years old, married with a grown-up family. She works part time as a clerical assistant. Mary consults her doctor because she is experiencing anxiety, depression, palpitations and urinary disturbances. The doctor diagnoses these symptoms as menopausal and prescribes a course of hormone replacement therapy (HRT), but to rule out the possibility of a urinary infection he asks Mary to take a midstream specimen of urine to the hospital pathology department. He also asks her to consult the practice nurse who will carry out further routine investigations. The practice nurse undertakes a nursing assessment. This involves interviewing Mary in order to:

1. Carry out routine investigations, i.e. weight, height, blood pressure and urine check (physical assessment);
2. Obtain information from Mary about her social and emotional health (psychosocial assessment).

As a result of this consultation Mary and the practice nurse may have identified the following concerns:

1. Mary is two stone overweight;
2. Mary feels lethargic for much of the time and is not sleeping well at night;
3. Mary feels very lonely.

Mary and the practice nurse can collaborate in order to plan a programme of care which may assist in alleviating some of these symptoms. It is likely that Mary will require the support of the practice nurse for a period of time as she becomes self-sufficient again, but during the course of this time the practice nurse may ask Mary to consult with the GP again if further medical intervention is thought necessary.

This scenario demonstrates how the roles of the doctor and the practice nurse differ, but complement each other. Nursing can extend and enhance medical care. Were Mary to undertake a course of HRT without nursing support it is possible that her symptoms may not improve, if only because she may not feel able to comply with the medical regime. This nursing assessment offers the following opportunities for health promotion.

- Access to a sympathetic listener;
- Examination of her lifestyle in relation to obesity and feelings of isolation.

In this respect therefore nursing can help the patient/client to come to terms with the social and psychological constructs of their medical problem.

The essential role of the GP is that of diagnostician and provider of the appropriate medical treatment. When an

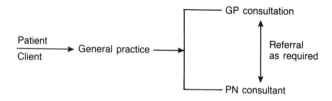

Figure 7.1 The relationship between doctoring and nursing in general practice.

individual feels unwell and visits their doctor they want to be told what is wrong and possibly to be prescribed some form of treatment, but any medical disorder is likely to carry with it social and emotional implications. Put simply we may feel unable to carry out our normal roles in life; psychologically we may feel depressed if we sense a lack of control. The practice nurse is the key person working in the surgery who can offer the patient this type of support and she may do this either directly or indirectly through various referrals.

Mackay concludes from the research results that both nurses and doctors have their own sphere of competence to which greater recognition needs to be given by the other. He argues that they need each other. The flow chart in Figure 7.1 illustrates how the relationship between doctoring and nursing could develop in general practice. It includes the notion of the practitioner concept of direct referral to the nurse if it appears to be appropriate.

Key points highlighted

- Doctors and nurses carry out roles which have evolved from different sociological perspectives. This clarifies some of the current problems concerning decision making and nurse autonomy.
- The notion of an autonomous practitioner in general practice is not yet a reality but there are features of the practitioner role that do equate to practice nursing which include:

- the extension of health education/teaching;
- the setting up and management of specific nurse run clinics;
- direct referrals to the practice nurse;
- the nursing diagnosis which takes into account the psychological and social dimensions of the medical disorder.
- In general practice there is interdependence between doctoring and nursing. Nursing can enhance health care for the practice population.

THE STRUCTURE AND CULTURE OF THE GENERAL PRACTICE ORGANIZATION

Many practice nurses will be familiar with the prevailing type of organization which generally operates in a large hospital setting where many levels of hierarchy exist. This type of structure emphasizes the importance of rules and procedures alongside the concept of subordination. The role an individual plays determines their status which in turn highlights the functional aspect of their job. Clark (1991) spells out the disadvantages of this 'role' culture in that it is not responsive to change and that the bureaucratic structure can decrease employee initiative.

The organizational structure of general practice is likely to be very different. Its small size means that it is possible for cultures to develop which do promote initiative and which are responsive to change in the environment. Many GPs have responded to various market changes quickly and this may in part be due to the lack of bureaucracy. Recognizing the type of structure and culture which is most prevalent in the practice can assist the practice nurse in health care planning. The following paragraphs delineate four different types of culture as described by Harrison (1972), cited by Handy (1984), and these cultures are discussed in their relationship to practice nursing.

Role culture

If this culture predominates, the role of the practice nurse is likely to be viewed in functional terms. Such a perspective helps the practice nurse to structure the workload accordingly. She has a clear job description and she is aware of what her role is and what is expected of her. She has little autonomy and little opportunity to implement new initiatives.

Power culture

If this culture predominates the central power source is all-important; this may be the senior partner in the practice who looks for trust and empathy with the emphasis on the importance of personal conversation as the main means of communication. The power culture is usually able to respond quickly to a changing market so that if extra nursing is perceived as necessary within the practice this would be initiated. There is emphasis on results and with much work being carried out with regard to audit, one can see that this culture may well be quite common in general practice. For the practice nurse this allows for various opportunities in that she is likely to enjoy a degree of autonomy and be encouraged to develop new initiatives especially if she can justify them by backing up any arguments with statistics.

Task culture

The practice nurse may be in a position to organize health care utilizing a team approach. Basically this type of culture looks to getting the job done by utilization of appropriate resources and expertise. Group power may improve efficiency and decision making occurs at grass roots level. Again this approach can be flexible to market changes and the practice nurse may enjoy considerable autonomy. She may initiate small scale research projects enlisting the co-operation of the administrative staff. She may carry out clinics in conjunction with the GP. Both of these are examples of work in a task culture organization.

Person culture

In direct contrast to the role culture, the person culture operates on the premise that the organization is subordinate to the person, the individual person being considered as a key element. Influence is shared equally and decision making rests with various individuals. Clark suggests that sometimes this culture can be seen within a larger organization and she refers to consultants working within the National Health Service who regard the organization as a base on which to further their interest and careers, both of which may indirectly benefit the organization. Some general practices may incorporate this type of culture especially if the GP has a particular research interest to pursue. A practice nurse operating in this type of organization would need to feel confident about decision making and to enjoy working on a 'practitioner' basis.

It is likely that the general practice organization will incorporate some of the features from these various cultures although on close examination one type may be dominant. It is generally recognized that the practice nurse role is diverse and that the job definition is likely to vary within different practice settings. For this reason it is valuable for the practice nurse to establish how the practice is structured and examine the prevailing culture because it is within this framework that health care will be planned. There is no one structure which is right or wrong and sometimes as goals change so will the structure. Within all these cultures, opportunities exist for the practice nurse to optimize health care, but the ideal practice structure is the one where a psychological match exists between the nurse and the practice.

Key points highlighted

- Practice nurses do not work in isolation but in relationship with other members of the general practice setting. There are many ways in which this setting may operate and the structure and culture of the organization provide the framework for the operationalizing of nursing care.
- Recognizing the prevailing culture can assist the practice nurse in planning nursing activities so that harmonious relationships with other members of the practice develop accordingly.
- The structure/culture is likely to change especially if the organization grows and takes on more complex technology.
- The practice nurse needs to feel comfortable or experience a psychological match with the prevailing culture in order to provide optimum health care.

A MODEL OF PRACTICE NURSING (FIGURE 7.2)

This model of practice nursing demonstrates the crucial role of assessment in nursing practice. Judgements are made and care planned accordingly; the practice nurse is continually making rapid judgements by the nature and number of interactions which normally occur throughout the day. The more information there is available concerning a patient/client, the more likelihood there is of an accurate assessment. The value of the assessment of the practice population as a whole has been referred to in an earlier chapter and information gleaned here may well provide the background for other assessments.

It has been established that assessments concern data collection but the crucial role of the practice nurse is to reflect on that data so that conclusions may be drawn from them. How does one fact relate to another? Is there, for instance, a direct relationship between an area of deprivation that exists in the local community and the number of people who consult the doctor? Do these people visit the surgery more frequently than another group of people? If the practice appears to have an increasing number of patients consulting with symptoms of

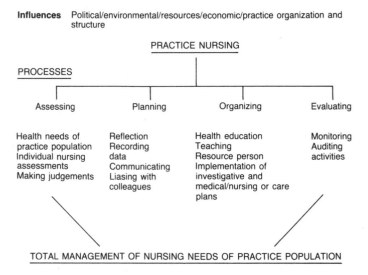

Figure 7.2 A model of practice nursing.

lethargy and depression, is this related to a characteristic which is occurring in the community? If a general practice has existed in the same place for many years it is likely that the pattern of consultations has mirrored the stresses faced by the community as a whole over that time. A practice profile offers the nurse a snap shot of a given period of time and this can serve as a baseline for planning future changes, because it can be used as a working tool.

An assessment may be assisted by use of a model, because it can provide a structure and afford a way of viewing a situation pictorially. It may form a broad picture which takes on board all the various components involved and so it offers a conceptual framework which encourages us to look laterally and take into consideration all the parts in relation to the whole. A model which appears to lend itself to the purpose of practice nursing is one proposed by Neuman (1980). Neuman's model is referred to as a systems model because primarily it describes a systems approach which suggests the following:

- There is a basic structure which is made up of several parts.
- There is a protective surrounding of the basic structure which is permeable.
- There is continual input data which may affect the basic structure.
- An output occurs after the process of adaptation in the basic structure.
- There is a feedback mechanism.

A simple systems diagram is illustrated in Figure 7.3.

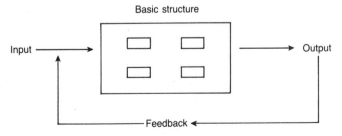

Figure 7.3 Outline of a systems model.

The systems approach can be applied to individual nursing assessments or to whole communities. Neuman describes her nursing model in the following way.

The basic structure is the individual's core and comprises various parts which relate to one another. These are the physical, psychological, social, genetic and cultural components of our being. We protect this basic structure by utilizing various lines of resistance and lines of defence and if these fail to operate then we are likely to suffer from a disorder. Examples of our protective ability could include our immune system or our coping mechanisms.

The input or the stressors which have affected our lifestyle may cause maladaptation to occur. Neuman suggests that we tend toward homoeostasis and seek to restore the imbalance wherever possible. Sometimes we are self-sufficient in that we restore the imbalance by treating ourselves if we are ill or we seek professional help.

Pearson and Vaughan (1986) offer a simplified version of Neuman's health care systems model which is depicted in Figure 7.4. Stressors are categorized in three ways:

- **intrapersonal** where the stressor is related to disease, infection or to specific life events such as grief;
- **interpersonal** where the stressor may be related to conflicts between people or within a family;
- **extrapersonal** where the stressor occurs outside the individual and could be related to various circumstances – financial, occupational, educational.

The practice nurse assesses the patient/client, keeping these categories of stressors in mind because the goal is to help the person toward maintaining the required balance. According to Pearson and Vaughan basically the nurse wants to:
1. prevent maladaptation occurring;
2. restore the adaptation;
3. maintain the adaptation.

These three interventions relate to primary, secondary and tertiary prevention. Primary prevention for Neuman is about identifying a stressor before it has actually caused a problem for the patient so that it can be dealt with. A simple example could be a weight reducing diet for an obese person or support

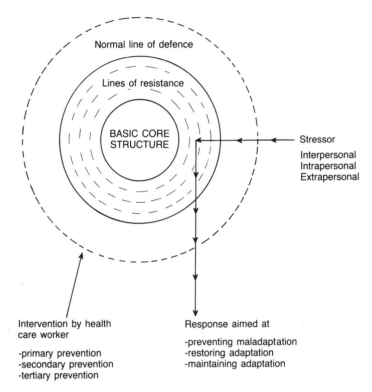

Figure 7.4 A simplified version of Neuman's health care systems model (reproduced with permission).

stockings to prevent varicose ulcers. Restoring the adaptation or secondary prevention is about providing the appropriate treatment which may be assisting in administering a course of drugs or dressing a wound. Maintaining the adaptation or tertiary prevention is about preventing any further maladaptation and involves making maximum use of all available resources. The practice nurse may not be able to cure asthma or diabetes but can perhaps ensure that its management is such that the balance is maintained as far as possible.

The assessment process can be facilitated, Neuman suggests, by using six basic questions:

1. What do you consider to be your major problem, difficulty or area of concern?
2. How has this affected your usual pattern of living or lifestyle?
3. Have you ever experienced a similar problem previously? If so, what was that problem and how did you handle it? Was your handling of the problem successful?
4. What do you anticipate for yourself in the future as a consequence of your present situation?
5. What are you doing and what can you do to help yourself?
6. What do you expect care givers, family, friends and others to do for you?

(Pearson and Vaughan, 1986)

The posing of these questions provides the framework which may assist the practice nurse in finding out from the patient and carer what are the main problems causing stress at this time. These can be discussed with the patient and then prioritized and categorized under the intra/inter/extrapersonal headings, taking the nurse's own perceptions into consideration. This data collection will allow the formulation of a plan of care which will focus around the three levels of prevention.

1. What can the nurse do either directly or indirectly to assist in alleviating stressors which pose a potential threat? Nurse action may involve referral to another health professional or the involvement of a local support group.
2. How can the practice nurse restore a stressor which is causing maladaptation? Nurse action may involve implementing a nursing treatment programme or referral to a GP for medical treatment.
3. How can the practice nurse help the person to maintain the optimum health that they have? Nurse action here may be the supportive role and involve health education and the monitoring of progress with regular follow-ups.

With practice, the nurse will write down the pertinent information. Initially it may take time to focus on the key issues and sometimes nurses utilizing nursing models often complain about the amount of paper work involved. However, this model can direct nursing practice and provide a framework for nursing assessments; it is up to each individual nurse to use it as a tool.

Neuman's model related to the practice population

If Neuman's model is applied to the practice population it could be said that the basic structure comprises;

- the people;
- the environment;
- housing
- culture;
- occupation and leisure opportunities.

This basic structure would be defended by lines of resistance and defence in that services are in situ which afford this population maintenance of healthy living. For instance social activities are available and accessible for the different age groups and provide the opportunities for social support. There is a good transport network; schools are in the vicinity and there are health services available. There is a general consensus of opinion that this practice population carries out daily activities without too many problems.

Stressors which may occur.

- an increase in unemployment;
- pollution of various kinds;
- the closing down of specific leisure amenities;
- proposals to build a motorway nearby;
- no more council accommodation planned;
- the closing down of a residential care home for the elderly;
- a steep rise in the cost of public transport.

Any of these stressors could have an adverse effect on the health of the basic community structure. Intervention at primary, secondary or tertiary level could involve:

- approaching the community health council with regard to the closing down of the residential care home;
- lobbying the local member of parliament with regard to the high unemployment figures;
- approaching local housing committees about the lack of housing;
- approaching environmental health regarding the pollution problems and the lack of leisure amenities;
- approaching social services regarding voluntary transport.

Although these interventions may not be specifically classed as 'nursing activities', nevertheless they could have a tremendous potential effect on the health of the practice population as a whole. If all community nurses became involved to some extent in these types of activities in order to promote overall health care, it is possible that this would be as effective as time spent carrying out specific health promotion clinics.

For Neuman the goal of the health professional would be maintaining the right balance of care and services within the community in order to avoid maladaptation. Such an approach requires a collective body who view primary health care as essential and who expect and encourage the local people to become involved in the planning of the services which are central to their health.

Planning

The next stage is that of planning health/nursing care either for a group of clients or for an individual. The collected data need to be considered carefully so that sensible decisions can be made concerning effective and efficient planning. Sharing ideas with professional colleagues could be valuable. Initiating self-help groups or screening programmes for the elderly could benefit from a multidisciplinary approach. There is some evidence from the literature that planning care for individual patients with their participation is more likely to lead to compliance.

Organizing

This is about operationalizing the care planning and many activities could emerge here. Proactivity as opposed to reactivity may offer the practice nurse opportunities for health education. Preparation for carrying out the required nursing or medical treatments may allow more time for patient contact. The management of clinics designed to fulfil a specific need is an example of this. Any equipment likely to be required is ready at hand and so there are less disruptions.

Evaluating

Practice nurses need to review the situation regularly. For individual clients this means collaborating with them about the effectiveness of the care they are receiving and if it is deemed appropriate to carry out a further assessment. As stated in a previous chapter, evaluating is about comparisons – is this clinic the best way to manage care for diabetic patients? How do we know? There is a need for constant questioning.

Key points highlighted

- An overall model of practice nursing offers a conceptual framework of how the role can be operationalized; the working constraints are acknowledged and the processes which lead to the management of nursing needs for clients can be specified by way of the activities involved.
- By thinking about the total nature of the practice nursing role various concepts emerge and links can be made which may clarify situations and aid understanding.
- Systems thinking in relation to the work situation and in relation to the clients living in the community offers the practice nurse opportunities for proactive planning which may assist in promoting harmonious relationships.
- The use of Neuman's model or possibly another nursing model can provide the practice nurse with a framework within which to plan and implement care. With practice its use can aid thinking in that the broad framework encourages the practice nurse to consider the patient's social, emotional and environmental parameters alongside the medical diagnosis. Lack of a structure and lack of direction for nursing practice could lead to ad hoc assessments which may not provide sufficient information from which nursing diagnoses can be made. There is also value in the sharing of perceptions in that two practice nurses working in the same practice and who assess clients utilizing a model are likely to aid the continuity of care and improve communication – both between themselves and with the clients as they begin to participate in the management of planning and the implementation of their care.

By relating practice nursing to the nursing process parameters it is possible to see how assessment, planning, organizing and evaluating feature as key concepts in the nature of the role both from a wide perspective in relation to the practice population and also from the individual nurse–client perspective. Neuman's model can provide a structure to assist in the assessment process so that this becomes manageable. This approach begins with the client – what are the problems as they see them? The practice nurse can develop these into categories and this assists in making a nursing diagnosis.

THE THINKING PRACTITIONER

Bransford and Stein (1984) emphasize five components of thinking which are applicable to a wide variety of situations. The first component is the identification of the problems followed by the ability to define and represent them with precision. In order to do this it may be necessary to break the problems down into sub-problems which are more manageable. Given a scenario of five GPs in a group practice who employ seven part time reception staff, a practice manager and two part time practice nurses, possible problems which may emerge could be:

- a lack of communication between all members of the practice;
- inadequate resources to meet the demands of health care for the practice population;
- low morale and high sickness rate among practice staff.

Taking the first problem, some of the sub-problems could be identified as follows.

- There are differences of opinion between the GPs which sometimes cause friction and conflict.
- The roles carried out by the receptionists are not clearly defined.
- The practice nurses never pass on information to each other or plan future work.
- There are no practice meetings organized.
- There is no one prepared to lead the practice team.

These are just a sample of sub-problems which may relate to the initial problem statement and perhaps if some of these could be addressed then the main problem may become less significant.

Once the sub-problems have been precisely identified the next stage to consider is the 'exploration of strategies' and this involves close examination of the problems bearing the following points in mind.

- There are likely to be many possible solutions for the same problem and it is valuable to consider any novel or unusual approaches.
- Each individual is likely to be biased according to their own personal preferences.
- Always remember to acknowledge that one's own understanding is limited.

Some of the possible strategies to solve the sub-problem regarding the lack of communication between the practice nurses could read:

- Both practice nurses increase their hours in order to have an afternoon together for liaison.
- Both practice nurses meet regularly in their own time.
- The work hours of the practice nurses are reorganized so that there is always a half hour overlap.
- One of the practice nurses takes on full time hours.
- Both of the practice nurses take on full time hours.
- Another practice nurse is employed whose hours dovetail with the first two in order to provide the necessary liaison.
- The roles of the practice nurses are so clearly defined that there is no need for communication between them, i.e. they work for specific GPs and care for a particular section of the practice population.
- The practice nurses utilize the computer, the telephone or writing pads for communication purposes.
- One of the receptionists takes on the liaison role between the two practice nurses.

This list is by no means exhaustive – 'brain storming' can offer all sorts of possible strategies, some of which may be totally unacceptable at the time, but the purpose of this exercise is to encourage lateral thinking and this can be creative and exciting.

The next stage in the thinking/problem solving process is to decide on a strategy and to act on it. Once that strategy has been in operation for a period of time it is then necessary to look at the effects and if these are undesirable then one can look again at the other pathways and implement another strategy. Bransford and Stein use a mnemonic for these five components which reads I D E A L.

Identify the problems.
Define and represent them with precision.
Explore the possible strategies.
Act on these strategies.
Look at the effects.

The value of establishing critical thinking nurses may well be reflected in the practical planning of care because thinking nurses will take account of the various ways in which the client views their situation and not be solely directed by the medical focus.

REFLECTIVE PRACTICE

Thinking is closely associated with reflection but for many nurses the focus is on continued action, leaving little room for the process of reflection. Hughes (1985) expresses concern in that the pressure to act tends to result in the perpetuation of traditional ways of giving nursing care and because of this pressure there is little opportunity for nurses of any grade to reflect on what they are doing.

Clarke (1986) explores that concept of action within the model of personal action proposed by the British psychologist John Shotter. Shotter (1975) refers to the person primarily as a doer who interacts with other people. He differentiates between being responsible for actions which involve the thinking process as opposed to the 'happenings' or 'events' which just occur. Clarke argues that the keystone to Shotter's view is this responsibility in that the action is chosen from amongst other actions because it is 'intended' and there is a reason for performing the action. One's actions must be informed with a knowledge of the situation in which one is placed and the kind of action required to modify it according to one's needs. For Shotter, practical activity is primary – theoretical activity may emerge from and may serve to modify it. In action, knowledge and movement are integrated: action is movement informed by knowledge.

It is interesting to note that reactive action, when reflected upon, can be used as a basis for future reasoned action. Clarke suggests that theory enables spontaneous performance to be given an intellectual basis which can be referred to in order to evaluate actions in terms of their significance to others. This constitutes a continual modification and correction of practice but it cannot be conducted by those with no experience of those practices.

The nature of practice nursing embodies a variety of experiences which may necessitate 'reaction' from the practice nurse in the context of the rapid making of relationships which incorporate a major part of the role. Shotter's theory of personal action discussed by Clarke suggests that experiences within practice nursing increase in value upon reflection as the significance of the initial action is explored. Reflection allows the practice nurse to consider why an event incurred a particular action and for Shotter any responsible action carries with it reasons or explanations.

Experiential learning

Much has been written about 'experiential learning' which can be described as learning that arises from practice and this concept supports the theories proposed by Shotter and Clarke.

Kolb (1984) refers to Lewin's notion of experiential learning which suggests that this is achieved via a four stage cycle. An immediate concrete experience is the basis for observation and reflection. These observations are assimilated into a 'theory' from which new implications for action can be deduced and these hypotheses then serve as guides in acting to create new experiences. For Kolb this cycle emphasizes two important points – one is that the immediate personal experience is the focal point for learning and the second is the value of the feedback mechanisms which involve problem solving processes to generate further information. The information feedback provides the basis for a continuous process of goal directed action and evaluation of the consequences of that action. This cycle of learning could be an invaluable aid for the practice nurse via the medium of a personal learning log. In order to incorporate this model into general practice the nurse can write regular entries into a personal learning log. This involves organizing set times during the week in order to record various happenings and events. The log can then be used as a basis for learning if the reflective process is utilized.

An example of entry in learning log

Thursday a.m.

Client Mr Jones and his wife visited for Mr Jones's final jectofer injection. No problems but just as they were leaving Mrs Jones sighs, 'Thank goodness the course is finished – now he will stop being sick as soon as we get home'.

Reflections

The practice nurse was particularly busy that morning and did not stop Mrs Jones to ask her what she meant by her comment. She now regrets this lack of action and begins to wonder if there is a connection between the sickness and the drug. If so, what are the implications of this? If the client is allergic to the substance what alternative treatment is available for him and will this allergy have caused physical harm to the client?

From this short and simple entry it is easy to see how much information may be learned from a concrete experience. Apart from information about the drug itself, adverse reactions and so forth, the practice nurse may want to consider how she should act should a similar situation arise. Her 'thinking' process may cause her to consider several areas of concern both about the involvement of the client in his treatment and about the management of the clinic if there is insufficient time for communication. The use of a personal learning log can aid learning on an informal basis and can be used as evidence of learning to attract academic credit.

Induction

Learning which emerges from practice can result in the formulation of specific explanations; practice nursing is a rich source of practice by definition of the job and nurses can capitalize on their experiences, using them as a basis for reflection and 'inductive reasoning'. Induction is considered to be a form of logical reasoning from which a generalization is induced from a number of specific observed instances. An example of this in general practice might be:

Observation All clients who appear to exhibit high levels of anxiety are unable to absorb health education concerning smoking, diet and exercise.

This is a specific statement which has arisen because of the practice nurse's observations and a generalization may be drawn from it which would read: 'Certain health education programmes are inappropriate for clients who are highly stressed'.

There is a school of thought which suggests that essentially nursing theory should emanate from practice and inductive reasoning could assist in this process. However, the information used in induction is based on the probability of observed cases and this does not necessarily establish truth or certainty because new circumstances could change the conclusion, but if the knowledge base for nursing could be developed or enlarged then this would appear to be a worthwhile activity.

Nurse theorists enjoy writing about how nursing ought to be and Miller (1985) confirms the view that practitioners need theory which they can relate to practice. For Miller, that theory needs to be narrow so that it can be usefully applied and she argues for a simple model which could be used for patients undergoing minor surgery. Is there a need here for a complex biopsychosocial approach? If Miller's argument is taken on board, there are many theories available which practice nurses could consider in relation to certain aspects of their work and examples of these could include:

- theories relating to personality and motivation, such as Maslow's hierarchy of needs;
- theories relating to communication and counselling;
- sociological theories relating to role and function;
- theories relating to stress, adaptation and coping;
- theories underpinning educational skills.

These 'narrow' theories could assist the practice nurse by providing an initial 'academic reference'.

Application of Maslow's hierarchy of needs for care of diabetic clients

Figure 7.5 illustrates the framework proposed by Maslow (1970). For nurses this could be a useful reference in that the framework is based on needs. Many nurse theorists have developed the concept of need and incorporated it into their nursing models. For instance, Roper refers to 12 activities of living and Orem describes self-care requisites which equate with needs.

Maslow proposes that human beings need to satisfy certain basic needs before they can proceed to satisfy other needs such as the need for affection and self-esteem. The idea of the pyramid shape is to demonstrate the importance of the needs in the lower segments. Much has been written about this hierarchy and there are arguments which suggest that human beings do not necessarily fulfil their needs in this order. For the practice nurse who is planning care for diabetic clients it could be a useful tool and the following case study attempts to show how the framework could be applied.

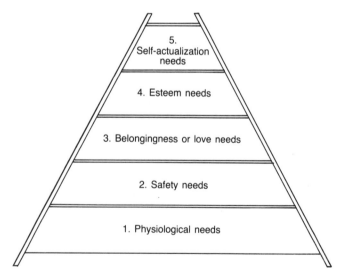

Figure 7.5 Maslow's hierarchy of needs ranges from the basic physiological needs, including hunger and thirst, to self-actualization needs, the highest needs (reproduced with permission from Maslow, 1970).

John, aged 36, is a school master, married with two children and has recently been diagnosed as diabetic. From the pyramid it can be seen that for the practice nurse and client the initial focus would be on the physiological changes which may have occurred as a result of the diabetes. The lower sections would also prompt the practice nurse to consider the 'safety' factors and for John this could include a number of issues. For instance does he understand the importance of a balanced diet which suits his lifestyle? Does he understand the possible complications that may occur and know what action to take if necessary?

Once the basic needs are met the practice nurse can move on to the psychosocial areas which appear higher in the hierarchy. It is as this stage, according to Maslow, that the practice nurse would initiate action concerning a teaching programme for John so that he can manage his own care efficiently and effectively. If this is successful this should result in an increase in both competency and self-esteem.

Maslow refers to self-actualization as the desire to fulfil one's potential and for John the diagnosis of diabetes may be a serious setback for him both professionally and personally; he may feel unable to aim for promotion at work or to continue with his hobbies. Following Maslow's hierarchy, once the former needs are met this would then be the time to address some of the 'growth' needs. John may express concern about his commitment to sport activities at school and feel unable to develop this interest and he may feel that it is inappropriate for him to apply for more senior posts. The role of the practice nurse here could be to encourage John to take his situation slowly and to allow himself time to adapt to the new circumstances before making further plans. Once his self-esteem returns and he feels competent in managing his diabetes, he may then feel confident to pursue other goals.

The hierarchy is not a rigid tool and it does not suggest any specific time frame; it is referred to here in order to indicate that there are many simple theories and models which can be utilized by nurses in various fields and for various reasons. Sometimes a theory can be modified to adapt to a different situation. Encouraging the relationship between practice and theory promotes competence and credibility. It sows the seeds for the development of the 'expert' nurse who is able to explain the 'why' underpinning the 'how'.

Benner (1984) insists that nurses can only be considered as expert practitioners if they can demonstrate a knowledge base commensurate with a smooth performance. As the process of observation and reflection becomes an accepted part of the practice nurse's role, so the expansion of knowledge could lead to the formulation of new nursing theory. This can only happen when nurses really think about the explanations which underpin their practice.

Key points highlighted

- Learning to think so that new ideas are generated can benefit the planning of care in general practice. It is very easy to accept the traditional methods as being the only course of action. Creative thinking can aid decision making and become a source of pleasure, especially if it is shared.
- If practice nurses can take the time to reflect on their practices they will accumulate much important information which can be used to develop and improve future practice.
- In order to aid in the reflective process, a learning log can be a valuable tool.
- Substantial learning and observation in practice could lead to an expansion of information which would in turn lead to an enlarged nursing knowledge base. Nursing theory based on inductivism could emanate from the general practice setting and this could be an interesting challenge for practice nurses.
- Simple models and narrow theory can provide a framework for the practice nurse which may be more appropriate than attempting to apply a broad abstract model to every situation.

CONCLUSIONS

This chapter has attempted to look closely at the dynamics of practice nursing. As a key member of the primary health care team, the practice nurse can greatly contribute to and enhance the health of the practice population. As this population becomes more demanding of services, so the role of the practice nurse is likely to become even more challenging. There is a need, therefore, for a critical examination of the role alongside professional colleagues and serious consideration of how nursing care can be operationalized and managed so that it is both efficient and effective.

REFERENCES

Benner, P. (1984) *From Novice to Expert: Excellence and Power in Clinical Nursing Practice*, Addison-Wesley, Menlo Park, California.

Bevis, E. (1982) *Curriculum Building in Nursing: A Process*, 3rd edn, C.V. Mosby, St Louis.

Bolden, K.J. and Tackle, B.A. (1989) *Practice Nurse Handbook*, 2nd edn, Blackwell Scientific Publications, Oxford.

Bransford, J.D. and Stein, B.S. (1984) *The IDEAL Problem Solver*, W.H. Freeman, New York.

Clark, J. (1991) *A Case Study of a Unit/Area of Practice*, Distance Learning Centre, South Bank Polytechnic, London.

Clarke, M. (1986) Action and reflection: practice & theory in nursing. *Journal of Advanced Nursing*, 11, 3–11.

Cumberlege, J. (1986) *Neighbourhood Nursing – A Focus For Care*, Report of the Community Nursing Review, HMSO, London.

De Young, L. (1981) *The Dynamics of Nursing*, 4th edn, C.V. Mosby, St. Louis.

DHSS (1990) *The New GP Contract*, HMSO, London.

Handy, C. (1984) *Understanding Organizations*, 2nd edn, Penguin, Harmondsworth.

Hobbs, R. and Stilwell, B. (1989) *Nursing in General Practice: Clinical Care, Book One*, Radcliffe Medical Press, Oxford.

Hughes, F. (1985) What do nurses do? *Senior Nurse*, 2, 18–19.

Kolb, D.A. (1984) *Experiential Learning: Experience as the Source of Learning and Development*, Prentice-Hall, New Jersey.

Mackay, L. (1992) Nursing and doctoring: where is the difference? in *Themes and Perspectives in Nursing*, (eds K. Soothill, C. Henry and K. Kendrick), Chapman & Hall, London.

Maslow, A. (1970) *Motivation and Personality* 2nd edn, Harper and Row, New York.

Miller, A. (1985) The relationship between nursing theory and nursing practice. *Journal of Advanced Nursing*, 10, 417–24.

Ministry of Health, Central Health Services Council Standing Medical Advisory Committee (1963) *The Fieldwork of the Family Doctor* (Gillie Report), HMSO, London.

Neuman, B. (1980) The Betty Neuman health care systems model: a total approach to patient problems, in *Conceptual Models for Nursing Practice*, 2nd edn, (eds J. Riehl and C. Roy), Appleton-Century-Crofts, New York.

Pearson, A. (1983) *The Clinical Nursing Unit*, Heinemann, London.
Pearson, A. and Vaughan, B. (1986) *Nursing Models for Practice*, Heinemann, London.
Reedy, B., Metcalf, A.V., de Rounaine, M. and Newell, D.J. (1980) The social occupational characteristics of attached and employed nurses in general practice. *Journal of the Royal College of General Practitioners*, **30**, 477–82.
Shotter, J. (1975) *Images of Man in Psychological Research*, Methuen, London.

8

Practice nursing: profession or occupation?

Milly Smith

INTRODUCTION

Practice nursing is one of nursing's newer branches and as such it is still very much in its formative stage. Roles, functions and delineation of responsibilities are still being explored and developed. The speed of growth has shaken the foundations of practice nursing and altered the course of its development. The whole remit of the practice nurse has changed since 1989 and it will continue to change as the implications of policy initiatives come into operation in general practice. It is not only the changes that have occurred in primary health care that influence practice nurses but also developments in nursing. These changes will involve all groups of community nurses in an evaluation of their respective roles. It will be necessary to realign and reshape traditional modes of practice to meet the changing trends in health care and the different demands that they impose on nurses.

This pattern of change and progression in practice nursing and nursing in general is nothing new. It presents a microcosm of the historical developments of nursing and indeed of any occupation that is dynamic and strives to move forward. Keeping abreast of current issues demands a continuous process of change and progression; this process has never been more in evidence in nursing than it is today. To have knowledge of the evolution of nursing facilitates the understanding of where nursing is and the events that have shaped the present position. That in itself might seem enough but much more important in the sequence of events is that some historical knowledge can help nurses to shape the future of the profession. To be able to influence professional growth it is necessary to have a sense of the long term development of nursing and recognize what has shaped its culture and continues to influence its aspirations for the future.

The term 'nursing profession' is frequently used; I have already used it in this introduction, though it is questionable how much its meaning is understood. In its historical development nursing has been through a process of professionalization. This has been brought about gradually and, for the majority of nurses, has passed unnoticed but it is a natural process that occurs as an occupation matures.

This chapter attempts to explore the issues that have influenced the development of nursing and determine the changes that have occurred in the occupational status of nursing that have moved it in the direction of a profession. Examination of these issues may help practice nurses to both identify and shape their role within health care.

HISTORICAL LEGACIES OF NURSING

Nursing has faced a long hard struggle to realize its aspirations of becoming a profession. It started from a point of anonymity and many historical influences have compounded and confused the issues.

The early Dickensian images of the Sarah Gamp type of nurse as drunken and slovenly are no myth. Pauper nurses were little better off than the paupers that they nursed and Louisa Twinning, in her report on asylums in the 1800s, observed that the nurses were not respected, had no authority in the asylums and consequently exercised control through bullying those under their care (Longmate, 1974). Not a particularly good starting point for the reputation of nurses.

Nurses lacked any sort of status and they were regarded in very much the same light as maids. A clear account of the position of nurses is given by Rosemary White (1978) in her work on the development of the nursing profession. She cites John South's description of the organization of a ward (1857). It portrayed the nurses as nothing more than ward maids and the sisters as their supervisors. The sisters had an additional role of administering the medicines, applying the poultices and feeding the patients. South, a surgeon at St Thomas's, affectionately portrayed them 'as if they were old superior family servants'. Once set, this image became a difficult one to shed.

Some nurses were not content with that position, the most well known being Florence Nightingale who strived to alter the demeaning position of nursing. She was the instigator of training for nurses and it was said of her that she improved the dismal reputation of nursing to that of an art (Leddy and Pepper, 1989). Florence Nightingale attempted to move to a position where nursing was managed by nurses. She held the view that nurses should be under the management of a trained female nurse rather than a doctor. This she achieved in part as her lady probationers moved out of the training schools and into major areas of the community though independence in nursing was never wholly achieved.

One of the factors that contributed to this, as Florence Nightingale recognized, was that nursing had two dimensions; the oldest role might be said to be that of caring for the patient and assisting their recovery, but the other dimension of the role was to assist the doctor. These two roles still remain today; they are distinct and yet interrelated. The assistant to the doctor implies a working partnership and the caring role is unique to the nurse. Some writers view the partnership role with medicine as one of subservience. Freidson (1970) was emphatic that all nursing and paramedic roles are by nature subservient to medicine because their knowledge and skills must be taught by or approved by physicians. This type of thinking may be one of the key issues that has thwarted the drive for full professional status. Nursing cannot be independent as a profession but that could also be said of medicine. Though the particular independent role that the nurse plays has been largely established there is duality and this can cause confusion where nursing autonomy is concerned.

That women ever went into nursing was a miracle; it was of low standing, poorly resourced, demanded long hours of duty and was regimented to the point where even relaxation hours and sleep hours were specified (Smith, 1982). These measures were probably necessary to upgrade the image but they took on an identity that started to shape nursing. Nursing for many years held on to the image of rule by senior nurses and physicians. Rule was by authority and demanded obedience; questioning or original thinking by learners and juniors was positively discouraged.

From these seemingly impossible beginnings the identity of nursing began to emerge. Once a nucleus of trained staff was established there was sufficient impetus to bring about change. One of the most influential effects of trained nurses was the notable improvement in standards of nursing care, both in the Poor Law infirmaries and the voluntary hospitals. Trained nurses were seen by the physicians to be more dependable and a marked improvement was noted in patient rehabilitation and the implementation of medical orders (White, 1978). 'Enthusiasm for the subject of nursing was at this time spreading rapidly' (Burdett, 1893). The value of nursing was beginning to emerge and show dividends in the contribution made to patient care.

Society was undergoing rapid changes, as has been noted in previous chapters. These developments greatly influenced medicine and nursing as they saw the dawn of anaesthetics, microbiology, X-rays and chemotherapy. As a result of these changes, nursing became established with doctors relinquishing work to nurses to free themselves for their clinical work and sisters gradually taking over the management of the wards. Nursing split, the Poor Law nursing retaining a traditional caring role with a more technical, medically orientated model being adopted by the nurses working in the voluntary hospitals. Divisiveness in nursing had a great influence on the progress of professionalization, an aspect developed later in the chapter.

More money was spent on nursing. Between 1860 and 1890 the cost of nursing quadrupled with the increased cost mainly due to improvements in working conditions in an attempt to attract the right calibre of person into nursing (White, 1978). The theoretical model as envisaged by Florence Nightingale, in which recognition was given to the importance of the environment of care, was beginning to pay dividends (Kjerwick and Martinson, 1979). By the middle of the ninteenth century nurses were providing value for money. Their contribution was reflected in the fall in the surgical death rate from 25–40% to 4%. This was largely as a result of the employment of aseptic techniques (Burdett, 1893). As the value of nursing became apparent so its development was established.

As nurses became established they grouped for strength and 1874 saw the foundation of the National and Metropolitan Nursing Association. Registration came much later in 1919. Though these small beginnings took many years to achieve they were the foundations of the professionalization of nursing, education, group identity and legislative recognition.

What is difficult to imagine is the enormity of the achievement. The cause was not won easily. The Victorian image of women, which had a strong influence on how women were perceived, was that of the weaker sex, fragile, prone to faints, mentally and physically inferior to men. Leddy and Pepper (1989) refer to the American woman as modest, humble, pious and chaste which no doubt provides an equally fitting description of the British female of that period. Women were supposed to find fulfilment through marriage and motherhood. Employment was not regarded as fitting or necessary for the majority of middle class women. They were generally powerless, were not expected to work, unless unmarried, were dependent on their husband for home and finance and were confined to a life of domesticity. They were not encouraged to move out of the circle of home and family and were thus restricted in their knowledge of the world about them. Angela Holdsworth (1988) refers to the position of women at this time as 'dolls in a doll's house' which seems to be an apt description.

The position for women who had to work was very different. The untrained working class were accepted into few positions: retail, clerking, factory labour, domestic service or prostitution (Bullough and Bullough, 1978). Women from the middle classes who had the benefit of some education found places as governesses and teachers. Nurses were generally recruited from unmarriageable middle and upper class women (Carpenter, 1977). Small wonder that they were submissive, willing to take orders from matrons and doctors and content to see nursing as an extension of domestic duties. Thus nursing became a refuge for substantial numbers of ladies who had been socialized into a lifestyle that was for the most part privileged and thrived on submissive obedience.

Times of great social change did eventually bring improvements for women. The suffrage movement fought for fairer recognition and opportunities. Women were able to operate in society in ways that were revolutionary and the more doors were opened to them, the more their work and capabilities were recognized.

The other major restraining factor of the time was the power of the medical profession. The history of medicine, however, has trodden a very different path. This chapter has already mentioned that physicians perceived nurses as the equivalent of a housemaid in the ward. The profession of medicine has roots that go back to the Greeks and Hippocrates, though some would suggest an even longer history (Sigerist, 1951). Freidson (1970) claimed that the true point of professionalism was realized in the late nineteenth century when the work of the physician became superior to that of other similar healers. The superiority arose from the establishment of medicine as a science rather than an art. Discoveries in medicine were underpinned by good education and university education was then a requirement for the practice of medicine. Freidson suggested that this placed medical practitioners in a position that was superior to other health practitioners who were operating much more from subjective rather than objective theories.

Once physicians reached the point where they held a body of knowledge that was unique, they were in a position where, in order to gain from that knowledge, the lay members of society had to consult them. This was a position of great strength and, once attained, was naturally jealously guarded. Physicians were in this position when nursing as a discipline was only beginning to emerge. The physicians of the late nineteenth century were working with nurses whose image has been typified in the earlier pages of this chapter. The marked difference in their position was established and continued through the next 100 years. Even today in both nursing and the paramedical services, the element that requires the physician to prescribe and delegate parts of patient care remains. This is the one feature that sustains the superiority of medicine over other health providers.

PROFESSIONAL DEVELOPMENT

As nursing set out on its road to becoming a profession, the legacies that shaped the early years were to stay with it for many more. The process of professionalization has been a long one and its principles will now be explored.

An interesting model of the professional growth of nursing has been suggested by Ainsworth-Land (1982) who offers the idea that nursing has moved through three stages. Stage 1 was that of informal apprenticeship where the role of the nurse was based on intuitive caring and experience. Stage 2, termed the normative stage, was the stage where nurses operated from a medical model of care. At this stage they had not clarified the concept of nursing sufficiently to be able to clearly differentiate nursing from the medical model and, more importantly, articulate the uniqueness of the discipline of nursing. Stage 3 of the Ainsworth-Land model, the integrative stage, is what nursing is striving to achieve. At this point education is university based, nursing is centred around its own paradigm, individual care is practised on a one-to-one basis with a team approach and there is a collaborative relationship with other health professionals.

It is probably fair to say that in the early 1990s nursing straddles the normative and integrative stages of this model. Some nurses have moved into the integrative stage and operate from a position where they feel that they are beginning to establish what nursing is all about. Others carry out a much more traditional approach to nursing and remain in the normative stage of the Ainsworth-Land model.

The next section of the chapter will explore how nursing has changed through its history, it will consider the key issues that have influenced development and will attempt to establish the current professional position of nursing. The starting point for the discussion will be an exploration of the concept of 'profession'.

Profession is a term that is used loosely in modern society. People may use the term 'professional' when referring to doctors, teachers, accountants, plumbers, secretaries. Advertisements refer to professional service, actors claim that they are professionals and prostitutes that they belong to the oldest of all the professions. None of these usages is incorrect and that suggests that there is no precise or absolute definition of the term. Cogan (1955) suggests that the term 'profession' has three uses. It may be used as a persuasive definition to imply high standards of service. It may be used as an operational definition to explain the organization and practice of a profession and it may be used as a logistic definition. In the logistic sense it attempts to describe historical connotations.

The original professions were more tightly defined and for many years portrayed a specific type of person. A professional in the preindustrial era was very definitely from the upper social classes, often the younger son who had no inheritance. The term was much more to do with position in society than any other feature that would be typically associated with the modern use of the term. The professions mentioned in the 1841 census were deemed to be the clergy, physics (physics denoting physician) and lawyers. By 1881 the list had grown to include solicitors, surveyors and the higher civil service (Baly, 1983).

The medical profession has often been cited as an example of a true profession. The original physicians who had to be educated through either Oxford or Cambridge universities actually had little medical teaching but rather concentrated on a classical education. Medical skills were gained following university education by either 'walking the wards' and observing or by attending private lectures from eminent physicians of the day (Newman, 1957). Gentlemanly manner, impressive behaviour and the client's ignorance were the foundations of medical practice. An appropriate picture is created by the words of Marshall (1939): 'The professional man does not work in order to be paid, he is paid in order that he may work'.

Industrialization brought a new era to professional practice. It removed it from the straightjacket of the class system (Marshall, 1939). Durkheim (1964) observed how economic activity became elevated with industrialization where formerly it was regarded as a minor and despised part of social life. Professional practice became associated with expertise and excellence and was firmly based on sound education. Rather than being associated with stasis and tradition it began to be seen as dynamic. Elliott (1972) suggested that professions at the end of the nineteenth century had two divisions, the traditional cultured gentlemanly lifestyle which contrasted with the changes that were determined by newfound knowledge, economic and social awareness.

Millerson (1964) described the process of professional development at this time as dynamic and operating on three different levels, the first being associated with the dramatic social change brought about by the post-industrial era, the second with the changing demands and aspirations of occupations and organizations and the third involving the ways that individuals adapt and operate in different professions. Millerson calls this the individual life cycle.

It seems that the concept of profession at that time was one of a service with the professionals as the sole providers of particular sets of skills that were required by the general population. Holding expert knowledge endowed professionals with autonomy and freedom in practice that was directly attributable to the influence and mystique that they had over lay members of society (Elliott, 1972). The professions became elite groups and their elitism was maintained by limiting the numbers who were admitted into the various professional groups. In this way their power and influence was reinforced.

This very traditional view that suggested that only the clergy, physicians, lawyers, surveyors and the higher echelons in the civil service were professionals has been challenged and largely replaced by one that considers that it is possible to move from occupational status along a continuum to professional status (Pavalko, 1971). The dramatic changes in social structure, technology and wealth distribution have seen the diminishing role of some of the older professions, particularly the clergy, while new services and industries have begun to fulfil the criteria that allow them to work towards professional status by changing the characteristics of their work.

Requirements of a profession

The modern concept of a profession incorporates the view that an occupation can move towards professional status as it becomes established and gains its own identity. The work of Pavalko (1971) on the occupation–profession continuum offers a concise account of the ways that occupations change and develop. As they do this so they adopt the characteristics of a profession. Pavalko's work was collated from a consensus of the key features that occur in the extensive literature on the subject of profession. According to Pavalko eight characteristics feature in the make-up of professional practice. They are identified in the following list.

1. Theory or intellectual technique
2. Relevance to basic social values
3. The training period
4. Motivation
5. Autonomy
6. Sense of commitment
7. Sense of community
8. Codes of ethics

The notion of an occupation–profession continuum suggests that some occupations, as they mature and change with time, move forward and adopt the characteristics of a profession. The characteristics are illustrated in Figure 8.1 at the two extremes of the continuum. At one extreme the characteristics are those that are related to an occupation, the other extreme illustrates those that would be associated with a profession. The notion of a continuum suggests that there is movement. Nursing is somewhere on the continuum.

Dimensions		Occupation		Profession
1. Theory, intellectual technique		Absent	_____	Present
2. Relevance to social values		Not relevant	_____	Relevant
3. Training period	A	Short	_____	Long
	B	Non-specialized	_____	Specialized
	C	Involves things	_____	Involves symbols
	D	Subculture unimportant	_____	Subculture important
4. Motivation		Self-interest	_____	Service
5. Autonomy		Absent	_____	Present
6. Commitment		Short term	_____	Long term
7. Sense of community		Low	_____	High
8. Code of ethics		Undeveloped	_____	Highly developed

Figure 8.1 The occupation–profession model (reproduced with permission from Pavalko, 1971).

The historic context of this chapter has attempted to establish the struggle that nursing had to reach the embryonic phase of development. The exploration that follows utilizes Pavalko's eight characteristics to explore the position that nursing has reached in the 1990s. Once the position of nursing in general has been assessed, the specifics of practice nursing may also be determined. The characteristics are discussed in the order that appears to develop the argument in the most logical manner.

The training period

From the early days nursing has been associated with an educational programme as a requirement for practice. Unlike medicine, nurse education has not been through the universities and has not resulted in a graduate workforce. Rather, nurse education has been a vocational education where a major service contribution has been linked with a programme of education. In this way the service side was often emphasized rather than basing the practice of nursing on a sound educational foundation. This type of programme is associated much more with an occupation than with a profession.

There have over the years been a number of educational milestones in nursing. Essentially there has been a gradual strengthening of the educational programme, which is consistent with professionalization. The change has occurred on several levels: the gradual increase in the length of the training programme, the developments of nursing knowledge, the increases in general knowledge about health and ill health, the progressive state of technology and research. All these factors have contributed to raising the level of nurse education to enable nurses to meet rising demands and expectations. This has been a long, slow process; some of the early reforms in nurse education go back to the 1940s.

The latest trends in nurse education were set in motion by the advent of Project 2000 (UKCC, 1987). This brave aspiration of the UKCC raised the quality of nurse education by not only setting the standard at a higher level, that of diploma instead of certificate, but also changing the status of nurses in training to that of true students. Nurses now learn to nurse in theory before they practise on people.

Project 2000 was only one move in the educational programme. What eventually emerged was a total picture where the educational experience can be conceptualized right through from student education to the stage of advanced practice. This total picture has been drawn through the amalgamation of several initiatives from the UKCC and national boards (Maggs *et al.*, 1990). The picture that emerges is one of initial preparation to the point of registration at diploma level (Project 2000), followed by consolidation of practice. Career progression will in future be achieved through a series of advanced programmes. These ideas were established in the following reports: *Post-Registration Education and Practice Project* (UKCC, 1989), *Community Education and Practice* (UKCC, 1991), The Higher Award (ENB, 1990). These programmes facilitate the move from diploma to degree and set an expectation that the specialist practitioner will be a graduate. An educational system such as this will inevitably result in nurses being educated to different levels. The idea of this was raised by Newman who uses the term 'tri-level system' (Newman, 1990). In this system nurses are used in three different ways: as professional nursing clinicians, as team leaders and as staff nurses. Newman equates each professional level with educational progression. In the British system the professional nursing clinician might hold a higher degree. The team leader might have a first degree and the staff nurse grades would occur from the point of registration which is currently diploma level.

The nature of this interlinked system is that it not only offers nurses clear guidance along the route for career development but, more importantly, the career development becomes dependent on education. In terms of professionalization this is a step in the right direction as it not only firms the educational basis of nursing but it also forces nurses to view education as a natural ongoing process throughout working life and one on which career aspirations are dependent. A hierarchical system such as this has the effect of creating an elite workforce which is in keeping with the concept of a profession.

Though the point of registration is not presently at graduate level the general move along the educational continuum is towards that eventuality. In this way the recent years have been crucially important to the professionalization of nursing.

Practice nursing is currently moving from a short ENB statement of attendance course towards the community health care nurse qualification. At the time of writing the level of this new course has not been established. It will be at a minimum level of diploma but is more likely to be a degree qualification. Practice nurses, along with school nurses, have further to move in their programme than other community colleagues whose courses have been at diploma level for some years. This anomaly illustrates the inconsistencies in the current system that expects qualifications at different levels for work that is essentially similar. The unfairness of this system has been a cause of controversy for many branches of nursing. For the first time in nursing's history there is a logical framework in place that clearly identifies the principles for career progression.

Theory or intellectual technique

Pavalko refers to this as 'the extent to which there is a sytematic body of theory and esoteric, abstract knowledge on which the work is based'. Pavalko goes on to offer medicine as 'an excellent example as its practice is based on the theory and research of anatomy, biology, chemistry, neurology'. In this respect medicine is fortunate in that the subject is very readily researchable and so the knowledge that is subsequently utilized can be scientifically based. This equally has become one of the criticisms of the medical model as the strength of the physiological sciences has overshadowed the influence on health of other potentially important areas, such as stress, housing and employment. The links between these were well covered by Illich (1977). He offered evidence that supported the fact that, historically, health gains were more influenced by socioenvironmental improvements than medical treatments. These issues have been slower to emerge from scientific research and they have largely been overshadowed by the medical model with its emphasis on diagnosis and treatment. Currently they are gaining acknowledgement as fundamental issues in health care.

The scientific knowledge base and the way it is utilized in nursing can be considered through examination of some of the areas that contribute to nursing practice.

Firstly, some of the knowledge base utilized by nurses is closely allied to medicine and over the years has been borrowed from the discipline. Medicine is by no means the only borrowed science; theories that focus on the social sciences of psychology and sociology have been drawn into nursing to contribute to the wider picture of factors that influence health and ill health and the understanding of the individuality of people.

Secondly, theorists have emerged from nursing. Florence Nightingale's *Notes on Nursing* (revised, 1970) offer some highly relevant observations and many of the principles remain as fundamental issues in nursing today. More recently, nursing academics have considered models of nursing in an attempt to clearly identify the uniqueness of the discipline. The contribution that academics have made has helped nurses to examine the concept of nursing and thus identify the features that are unique to nursing. Nursing theorists have helped to move nursing forward; thus, the firmer the nursing knowledge base becomes, the less nurses have to rely on the medical model of care.

Thirdly, over recent years the amount of original research that has come from nurses has grown. This may be attributed to the academic progress made by many nurses following registration. As the number of nursing degree programmes specifically designed for nurses has increased so knowledge and interest in research improves. Nurses become involved in research and this enlightens nurses' knowledge about nursing. This process sets into motion a circle of knowledge production. It seems that once the momentum is started it becomes self-perpetuating as one set of research findings provokes further questions that require investigation (Gruending, 1985).

Fourthly, the scientific basis of care has undoubtedly benefited from the research done by the pharmaceutical companies. Though the concept of vested interest should always prevent the blanket acceptance of product claims, there is no doubt that competition amongst companies has considerably improved both products and the evidence offered in their support. This improved area of knowledge covers issues that are at the core of nursing – wound care, pressure area care, rehabilitation, etc. Product research has greatly benefited nursing and enthusiastic marketing tactics have really raised awareness of research based practice among nurses.

The evidence that underpins nursing practice is available and increasing. What is questionable in this debate on professionalization is how much of the research evidence has emerged from nurses and, more to the point, how many nurses actually practise from a theoretical perspective. The answer to both those questions would be difficult to ascertain; perhaps the best that can be said is that there is a constantly increasing body of knowledge and that nurses are becoming more orientated towards its use.

Autonomy

Autonomy in practice means that the individual has the freedom and authority to act independently (Leddy and Pepper, 1989). The historical position that placed nurses in a subservient role to medicine would suggest that nursing can have little claim to autonomy. It is also suggested that nurses cannot be independent practitioners while they are employed by organizations who determine their role. The employer will naturally place constraints and choices on the scope of employment and within these restrictions nurses cannot be said to be autonomous practitioners (Copp, 1988). The general practitioner employs practice nurses which automatically implies that some form of management control is exercised and that practice nurses are not autonomous.

The organizational culture of general practice normally affords a degree of flexibility and this is one of the attractions of working in the general practice setting. Health authority employed nurses can be in a more invidious position as they are a part of a much larger bureaucratic structure where there are very formal rules and regulations that surround nursing practice. Rules are intended to protect employees but as they serve this protective function so in this particular argument they also place restrictions on autonomous practice. NHS management changes have increased the number of nonnurses in management positions, which in turn reduces the influence the nurses have over nursing. Restrictions placed on practitioners can be very constraining, particularly in the NHS, and the growth of practice nursing has been attributed in part to the restrictions placed on district nurses who were attached to general practices which prevented them from fulfilling the roles that the general practitioners thought appropriate for practice nurses (Bolden and Takle, 1990).

A further body of opinion suggests that nurses cannot be autonomous practitioners while they are in a position where some of their work is prescribed by doctors as this does not constitute autonomous practice, but there is also some suggestion that doctors are becoming deskilled. Larkin (1983) makes the point that nursing and paramedical staff are presenting a challenge to medical dominance; he attributes this to improved educational preparation which underpins their skills and at the same time builds confidence. The situation has undergone some improvement over recent years. By attempting to define and establish the concept of nursing, nurses have developed models that clearly delineate the role of the nurse from that of other health workers. In this way White (1988) suggests that nurses are attempting to shift the balance of control towards that of power sharing. Power sharing fits into the integrative stage of the Ainsworth-Land model and helps to support the idea that nursing is in part in the stage where working relationships are collaborative with other professionals.

Bernhard and Walsh (1990) hold the view that nursing autonomy is increasing but they offer a different concept of autonomy in which they suggest that autonomy occurs whenever nurses make clinical judgements about patients' problems. This suggests that autonomy does not have to encompass all aspects of practice but rather occurs where one practitioner holds the balance of expertise over another. Utilization of the concept in this sense requires that the same view is held by all contributors. At this time it is unlikely that it would be accepted by all nurses and even more unlikely that the medical profession would acquiesce to the idea.

Though there are serious concerns over nurses' degree of autonomy of action, it is encouraging that some trends in nursing are moving towards greater autonomy. Support has come from the UKCC in the form of the position statement in *The Scope of Professional Practice* (1992) where judgements about the scope of nursing practice are left to the individual practitioner to decide, using the Code for guidance. Other moves that have helped to promote autonomy have been the establishment of nursing standards. These codes of practice have provided nurses with a tool that can be used in peer evaluation, which Bernhard and Walsh (1990) claim is another move towards autonomy in practice. It negates the need for practice to be evaluated by non-nurses thus affording greater autonomy.

Code of ethics

Possession of a code of ethics is one of the marks of a profession. Probably the best known code is that of the medical profession, the Hippocratic Oath. What is the significance of a code of ethics? A code sets a level of acceptance and expected professional standards. Each member of the profession is expected to uphold the standards and sanctions can be taken against members who fail to comply. The code is set by the discipline that it regulates.

A code of ethics, as the name suggests, is a collection of standards that focus on expected behaviours. The code guides its members and helps them to judge acceptable professional behaviour for themselves and their peers. The nature of such a code is that it is often grounded on ethically based statements, though this is not necessarily the case (Burnard and Chapman, 1991). Thiroux's set of principles gives an indication of the issues that are involved in ethics. They are the value of life, goodness or rightness, justice or fairness, truth telling or honesty and individual freedom (Thiroux, 1980). It is easy to see how they can be embodied into a code of professional standards. It is also easy to see why a discipline such as nursing that involves so much trust and confidence should have such a code.

Nursing has had a written code of professional conduct since 1984 when the Nurses Act was revised. Prior to the written Code there were acknowledged acceptable standards of practice that were upheld through a disciplinary committee. Then, as now, nurses had to be registered to practise and those who were disciplined through the General Nursing Council disciplinary committee could face the ultimate sanction of having their name removed from the Register of Nurses. The code was unwritten but it existed.

The formalizing of the Code of Professional Conduct came with the revision of the Nurses and Midwives Act and the United Kingdom Central Council. The Code has undergone several revisions, the latest one being in 1992 (UKCC, 1992). Essentially the Code makes nurses, midwives and health visitors responsible for their actions. It does so through clauses which set the expectations for professional behaviour. Each person who is registered with the UKCC is sent a personal copy of the Code and thus should be fully cognisant with its content. The whole notion of the Code of Professional Conduct is that it has serious connotations and implications but for all this it is not law, it is there for professional guidance. This seems anomalous and has over recent years been the cause of confusion and frustration to nurses. It is difficult to appreciate why, under the Code, nurses can be disciplined for infringements but not adequately supported if they make a stand against practices that they feel are unacceptable. Derek Owen, a psychiatric nurse who made a stand against administering electroconvulsive therapy to a patient, was dismissed from his employment (Copp, 1988). Graham Pink, who complained that the staffing levels on night duty on an acute geriatric ward were unacceptably low, was also dismissed (Turner, 1992). It is intriguing that in neither of these incidents was the Code of Professional Conduct able to support the actions of the nurses. This suggests that the Code is rather one-sided – it places rights and duties on nurses but lacks supportive power due to its non-legal status.

The links between the Code of Professional Conduct and accountability are strong and this may cause serious moral dilemma for nurses who have to consider two masters with different sets of expectations, the Code with its moral and ethical obligations being one and the employer who is operating with increased demands and reducing resources being the other. Armstrong (1987) acknowledges that the UKCC Code is unclear and that controversy may weaken its claim to be a useful tool in the accountability of nurses.

The possession of a code of ethics or in this case a code of conduct is one of the areas of professionalization but it seems that the influence of the Code is stronger on nurses than it is on their employers. This could be a measure of the weakness of the professional position that nursing holds or it could be an indication of more fundamental changes to the role of professionals, in that judgements that for years were sacrosanct are being constantly challenged and overruled.

Sense of community

Community is used in this instance to suggest fraternity or oneness. It is suggested by Johnson (1989) that the sense of community is a continuous and terminal state that is shared by all members. The sense of community gives identity to the group; some of the ways in which this is fostered are through common education programmes, close supervision through an apprentice system and a developed network of communication through meetings, journals, books and a highly developed language or jargon. These are characteristics that are certainly recognizable in nursing but there is more to the sense of community and that is to do with the core meaning of life being central to the work situation. King (1968) refers to this as 'complete identity'. Nurses seem to fall short of this ideal.

The sense of community can be a powerful political tool for professional groups, as the General Medical Council demonstrates on behalf of doctors. Nursing does not hold this strong sense of community and loses power because it diffuses potential strengths by being politically naive and fragmented in representing its views. Fragmentation is demonstrated in the way that nurses use several trade unions and representative bodies, rather than speaking with one voice. It is also very apparent through the apathy that can prevail when disputes occur within the organization.

A strong sense of community can develop a protectionist attitude towards the profession. This in turn may lead to the formation of a monopoly where the services provided by a discipline are only available through the discipline. To hold a true monopoly nursing must be the only discipline that is eligible to provide nursing care. It has taken many years for nurses to decide what the concept of nursing actually involves, let alone to become the only provider of the service. It is only in comparatively recent years that nursing academics have explored the concept sufficiently thoroughly to be able to determine the key elements of nursing. This at least has enabled nurses to identify their own uniqueness and delineate their role from that of other medical and paramedical services. Understanding the concept does not of itself afford it a monopoly position. Rather, nurses have been willing to give away their traditional role to unqualified staff while they expanded the medical aspects by absorbing more of the technical work that has traditionally been within the remit of the medical profession.

In the 1990s a new challenge has emerged in the guise of skill and grade mix. Matters of economy are forcing managers to consider the employment cost of nurses, especially those in the higher grades. The fact that skill mix is being introduced by management makes it obvious that nurses do not hold a monopoly position; if they did it would be the nursing profession that directed the changes according to perceived needs that were based on professional judgements.

Even in the traditional professions, true monopolies of service may be heading for extinction; people other than doctors now diagnose and prescribe some treatments, including nurses when the Nurse Prescribing Bill (1989) is enacted (DHSS, 1989). Lawyers do not hold absolute monopoly; people can defend themselves in a court of law and estate agents carry out conveyancing on properties. As the world becomes even more complex the demand for more specialized and new skills grows and it becomes difficult for any one professional to hold the knowledge that encompasses such diversity. Professions cope with this by specialization and by shedding parts of the role. Reskilling and deskilling are terms used by Larkin (1983) who suggests that they may both be occurring at the same time as fewer of the fully qualified control an increasing number of lesser paid and trained aides. As this trend develops the question of any profession holding absolute monopoly status is questionable.

Sense of commitment

Commitment to the profession implies a lifelong commitment in that once accepted into a profession, it is unusual for a member to leave. This is not the case for nurses. Moloney (1992) suggests that most nurses stay in nursing for relatively short periods of time, viewing it as a temporary job rather than a fulltime career. This can be in part attributed to the largely female labour force and the consequent roles of wife and mother that impinge on career development.

Sense of commitment ought to be a historical concept that is becoming outmoded; it has connotations of male dominated professions which one would like to think are less of a feature of modern society. Career breaks ought to be the norm for young professionals but reality suggests that this is not possible for the majority.

Relevance to basic social values

This concept on Pavalko's list is one in which nursing can claim to be strong. The idea suggests that a profession places emphasis on improving the basic values of the field in which it operates, which for nurses is health. The tradition of nursing has been one of service, that is, person centred, rather than one which is profit orientated but this notion can cause conflict between managers and nurses in the current resource limited climate, particularly where decisions may not seem to be in the best interests of the clients.

The contributions that nurses make to health may be the ones that offer the broader view, one that encompasses the individuality of the person as well as the presenting health problem and then attempts to address the full picture in any interventions.

The concept of relevance to social values is an interesting one that may itself require examination. It does seem to suggest that no one whose occupation, no matter how worthy, does not contribute to social values can be considered a professional. Some sectors, for example manufacturing industry, may well hold the making of profit as the main objective but the fact that they create employment adds to social values, albeit indirectly. The importance of employment to a person's morale and self-image has become very evident in the current economic climate and if profit oriented organizations contribute to well-being indirectly, it could be argued that they contribute to social values.

Motivation

The desire to work for the benefit that it affords the client rather than the rewards that are personally accrued suggests that this is another area where nursing scores well. This again has been a part of the ethics of nursing; the adage that 'nurses are born and not made' supports the traditional view, which is largely also the current view. Whether this will change in relation to trends in society, particularly un-employment, remains to be seen. The difficulties that are presented to young people who are seeking work may mean that men and women enter nursing just to get a job and the question of motivation for the work could be subject to change. Time will tell.

Motivation towards the job and its relevance to social values appear to have close links and it may be that both are experiencing change in nursing that has been imposed by more general movement in society.

The occupation–profession continuum provides a framework for the examination of the position of nursing. It is apparent that some of the dimensions of the model are more developed in nursing than are others. In some dimensions such as theoretical and intellectual techniques, there has been advance-ment; in other areas such as autonomy there has been little development. It will be interesting to note the changes over the next few years to see where progression or regression occurs.

CONCLUSIONS

It is clear to see how loosely the terms 'profession' and 'professional' are used and how little they are understood. The traditional professions really were rooted in history and as such they had a distinct advantage as they gained power through monopoly over services and through the exclusivity that was maintained over entry to the profession.

Historical events may have initiated the professions but they also were the cause of their undermining for, as times and circumstances changed, so have demands. From the demands of the Industrial Revolution emerged new occupations. These occupations became more competent and more enlightened and eventually many of them held aspirations for professional status. Thus the traditional view of profession and professional was challenged and replaced by one that acknowledged the need for a more dynamic developmental approach rather than one that was static and protectionist.

Just as history shaped other professions so it shaped nursing by placing its origins with women and the caring role and allied to the dominant role of medicine. It has taken nurses many years to establish the identity of nursing and begin to provide the underpinning that nursing required before it could lay claim to the professional title.

The complexity of current health care provision has prompted many changes. There have been shifts in health policy to change the emphasis from hospital to community care, from dependence on the welfare state to a return to self-sufficiency. The organization of the National Health Service has undergone major changes that have diminished the power of the professional by strengthening the autonomy of managers. Health care has become increasingly complex and technical and the providers of care have taken on the challenge and gained expertise that is appropriate to contend with the demands. Today's developments are impacting on nursing and continue to shape its claim to professional status. Some of the dimensions of the Pavalko model of professionalization are closer to attainment while it is possible that other areas are being eroded.

Practice nursing as a branch of nursing was a late starter in as much as the shaping of its own identity was concerned. Naturally the general attributes of the nursing occupation/ profession were set during the nurse training. These would have been further influenced by post-registration experience and brought into practice nursing to provide the foundation on which to build. Subsequent influences that involve the very different role played by practice nurses and the fact that there is for most practice nurses an element of professional isolation are likely to have affected the shape of professional progress. The most positive outcome of this may be that it created a degree of self-sufficiency among practice nurses. Because of the tendency towards isolation from other nurses, practice nurses became adept at seeking information and identifying valuable resources. In this way the autonomous focus of the role was fostered and may well become more developed than would be the case in other working environments.

Another major influencing factor for practice nurses is their employment status, with the general practitioner being the employer. The general practitioner will naturally hold medical values and this may give rise to professional conflict. Nurses in this situation are bound by their code of conduct and as such are answerable for their professional actions. They are also answerable to their employer who may operate to a different set of professional medical standards that may not equate with nursing accountability. In this type of instance the practice nurse could well be on a different stage of the occupation–profession continuum, further along than most nurses in some ways and in others further back, having lost some autonomy to their employer.

Reflective exercise

Now that you have read this chapter it would be a good exercise in reflection to think about your own professional status. The headings used in the chapter are offered below as an aide memoire. As you determine your position on the occupation–profession continuum think about how you would justify your decisions. This will not be a quick or easy task but it may help you to identify your own personal and professional strengths and weaknesses. Determination of these is beneficial in several ways: it enables you to capitalize on strengths and build on weaknesses which can be seen as a move towards professional growth. Identification of nursing as a profession also helps to envisage the perceptions that other professionals may hold of nurses and nursing. This particular knowledge can prove invaluable in working relationships.

Being a member of a profession, as this chapter has illustrated, has important implications and there is far more to the concept than most people realize.

Where do you think practice nursing fits on Pavalko's occupation–profession continuum? Work through the headings in your own mind and mark the place on the lines below.

	Occupation	Profession
Theory, intellectual technique		
Relevance to social values		
Training period		
Motivation		
Autonomy		
Commitment		
Sense of community		
Code of ethics		

Is practice nursing at the same stage of development as nursing in general or is it further forward in some areas and further back in others?

REFERENCES

Ainsworth-Land, G. (1982) *Forward to Basics*, DOK, Buffalo, NY.

Armstrong, M. (1987) Contemporary ethics. *Nursing*, 3(14), 518–20.

Baly, M. (1983) *Professional Responsibility*, 2nd edn, John Wiley, Chichester.

Bernhard, L. and Walsh, M. (1990) *Leadership, the Key to the Professionalisation of Nursing*, 2nd edn, C V Mosby, St. Louis.

Bolden, K. and Takle, B.A. (1990) *Practice Nurse Handbook*, 2nd edn, Blackwell Scientific Publications, Oxford.

Bullough, V. and Bullough, B. (1978) *The Care of the Sick: The Emergence of Modern Nursing*, 3rd edn, Prodist, New York.

Burdett, H. (1893) *Hospitals and Asylums of the World*, Vol III, J. & A. Churchill, London.

Burnard, P. and Chapman, C.M. (1991) *Professional and Ethical Issues in Nursing, The Code of Professional Conduct*, John Wiley, Chichester.

Carpenter, M. with Stacey, M. (ed.) (1977) *Health and the Division of Labour*, Croom Helm, London.

Cogan, M. L. (1955) The problems of definitions and profession. *Annals of American Academy of Political and Social Science*, 397, 105-11.

Copp, G. (1988) Professional accountability: the conflict. *Nursing Times*, 84(43), 42-4.

DHSS (1989) Report of the Advisory Group on Nurse Prescribing, HMSO, London.

Durkheim, E. (1964) *The Division of Labour in Society*, Free Press, Glencoe, Illinois.

English National Board (1990) *The Framework and Higher Award for Continuing Professional Education for Nurses, Midwives and Health Visitors*, ENB, London.

Elliott, P. (1972) *The Sociology of Professions*, MacMillan, London.

Freidson, E. (1970) *Profession of Medicine: A Study of the Sociology of Applied Knowledge*, Dodd Mead, New York.

Gruending, D. (1985) Nursing theory, a vehicle for professionalisation. *Journal of Advanced Nursing*, **10**, 553–8.

Holdsworth, A. (1991) *Out of the Dolls House*, BBC Books, London.

Illich, I. (1977) *Limits to Medicine*, Penguin, Harmondsworth.

Johnson, T. (1989) *Professions and Power*, Macmillan Education, Basingstoke.

King, M.D. (1968) *Science and the Professional Dilemma* (ed. J. Gould), Penguin Social Science Survey, Harmondsworth.

Kjerwick, D.K. and Martinson, I.M. (1979) *Women in Stress: A Nursing Perspective*, Appleton-Century-Crofts, New York.

Larkin, G. (1983) *Occupational Monopoly in Modern Medicine*, Tavistock Publications, London.

Leddy, S. and Pepper, J.M. (1989) *Conceptual Basis of Professional Nursing*, 2nd edn, J.B. Lippincott, Philadelphia.

Longmate, N. (1974) *The Workhouse*, Temple Smith, London.

Maggs, C., Rogers, J. and Shuttleworth, A. (1990) *Framework for Continuing Professional Education*, ENB, London.

Marshall, T. H. (1939) The recent history of professionalism in relation to social structure and policy. *Canadian Journal of Economics and Political Science*, **5**, 325.

Millerson, G. (1964) *The Qualifying Associations*, Routledge and Kegan Paul, London.

Moloney, M.M. (1992) *Professionalisation of Nursing: Current Issues and Trends*, 2nd edn, J.B. Lippincott, Philadelphia.

Newman, C. (1957) The Evolution of Medical Education in the 19th Century, Oxford University Press, London.

Newman, M.A. (1990) Towards an integrative model of professional practice. *Journal of Professional Nursing*, **6**(3), 167–73.

Nightingale, F. (1970) *Notes on Nursing*, 2nd edn, Duckworth, London.

Pavalko, R.M. (1971) *Sociology of Occupations and Professions*, F.E. Peacock, Itasca, Illinois.

Sigerist, H. (1951) *A History of Medicine*, Vols I and II, Oxford University Press, New York.

Smith, F.B. (1982) *Florence Nightingale: Reputation and Power*, Croom Helm, London.

Thiroux, J.P. (1980) *Ethics, Theory and Practice*, Glencoe Publishing, Encino, California.

Turner, T. (1992) The indomitable Mr Pink. *Nursing Times*, **88**(24), 26-9.

UKCC (1987) *Project 2000: The Final Proposals*, UKCC, London.
UKCC (1989) *Post Registration Education and Practice Project*, UKCC, London.
UKCC (1991) *Report on the Proposals for Community Education and Practice*, UKCC, London.
UKCC (1992) *Code of Professional Conduct*, 3rd edn, UKCC, London.
UKCC (1992) *The Scope of Professional Practice*, UKCC, London.
White, R. (1978) *Social Change and the Development of the Nursing Profession*, Henry Kimpton, London.
White, R. (1988) *Political Issues in Nursing*, Vol 3, John Wiley, Chichester.

Index